TRANSCULTURAL COMMUNICATION
IN NURSING
Second Edition

D0290826

Dedication

*In loving memory of my husband, Jaime Y. Muñoz,
and in thanksgiving for my children, Carlo and Erica*

—Cora Muñoz

TRANSCULTURAL COMMUNICATION

IN NURSING

SECOND EDITION

Cora C. Muñoz, PhD, RN
Joan Luckmann, MA, RN

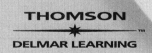

THOMSON

DELMAR LEARNING

Australia Canada Mexico Singapore Spain United Kingdom United States

THOMSON

DELMAR LEARNING

Transcultural Communication in Nursing, 2e
by Cora C. Muñoz, PhD, RN, and Joan Luckmann, MA, RN

**Vice President,
Health Care Business Unit:**
William Brottmiller

Editorial Director:
Cathy L. Esperti

Acquisitions Editor:
Melissa Martin

Editorial Assistant:
Patricia M. Osborn

Production Editor:
Anne Sherman

Marketing Director:
Jennifer McAvey

Channel Manager:
Tamara Caruso

Library of Congress Cataloging-in-Publication Data
Muñoz, Cora C.
   Transcultural communication in nursing / Cora C. Muñoz, Joan Luckmann.—2nd ed.
      p. ; cm.
   Rev. ed. of: Transcultural communication in nursing / Joan Luckmann. c1999.
   Includes bibliographical references and index.
   ISBN 0-7668-4877-9 (alk. paper)
      1. Communication in nursing—Cross-cultural studies.
2. Transcultural nursing. 3. Nursing—Social aspects.
4. Interpersonal communication—Cross-cultural studies.
I. Luckmann, Joan. II. Luckmann, Joan. Transcultural communication in nursing. III. Title.
   [DNLM: 1. Transcultural Nursing. 2. Communication. WY 107 M967t 2005]
RT23.L83 2005
610.73—dc22
                                                      2004051719

INTERNATIONAL DIVISIONS LIST

NOTICE TO THE READER

CONTENTS

PREFACE

This book, *Transcultural Communication in Nursing*, second edition, is designed for all health care providers and students in the helping professions. Anyone who interacts with culturally diverse patients and families needs to learn transcultural communication principles and techniques. In this society, with its continually changing racial, ethnic, and cultural demographics, opportunity for intercultural communication has accelerated. The globalization of the economy, new technology, changes in immigration patterns, threats to our homeland security, and other factors have contributed to the heightened interest in effective interactions and communication among groups from various cultural backgrounds. This practical book, although focused on nursing practice, has content that is highly relevant to the practice of all helping professionals working with culturally diverse clients and their families.

Increased demands for transcultural communication skills in nursing are apparent, and lack of awareness and knowledge about interacting with diverse groups and understanding cultural beliefs, values, and practices has created stress and frustration for the health care provider. Basic communication concepts and well-developed transcultural skills in communication can enhance the quality of health care services, address the barriers that can lead to poor care, and increase a sense of competence and satisfaction for the provider.

Nurses plan their care on the basis of the holistic needs of the client and families. This perspective recognizes the importance of incorporating cultural values, beliefs, practices, and communication patterns that can facilitate therapeutic relationships. This book discusses how transcultural communication concepts and principles are important in gathering assessment data, developing culturally appropriate nursing diagnoses, and implementing quality care.

Among the recommendations of the Institute of Medicine report on unequal treatment regarding racial and ethnic disparities in health care are recommendations to enhance patient–provider communication, support the linguistic needs and use of interpretation services, and integrate cross-cultural education and training. It is also noted in this report that language barriers pose a significant problem in accessing health care and can affect compliance to treatment regimes, appointment attendance, and levels of satisfaction with health care services. This book will enable readers to learn communication styles and patterns that will enhance their nursing skills to communicate with patients and families effectively. The chapters on transcultural communication barriers and working with and without an interpreter address some of the IOM recommendations.

The new guidelines from the Department of Health and Human Services on Culturally and Linguistically Appropriate Standards are incorporated in a new chapter of this textbook. This will provide the readers understanding of the expectations regarding care for persons with limited English proficiency. This content clearly complements the information on the use of interpreters and guides the organization to provide culturally appropriate services.

ABOUT THE AUTHORS

Cora C. Munoz, PhD, RN, is an immigrant from the Philippines who came to the United States 34 years ago, has genuine interest in and commitment to advancing cultural competence and transcultural communication. Through her experience of working with a diverse client population at Columbia Presbyterian Medical Center in New York City, she realizes the importance of cultural sensitivity and understands clients' varied cultural and linguistic backgrounds.

Joan Luckman, MA, RN, grew up in Los Angeles and received her basic nursing education at Los Angeles County General Hospital, where she learned about transcultural communication through first-hand experience with clients from dozens of insular racial and ethnic neighborhoods.

ORGANIZATION AND CONTENT

Transcultural Communication in Nursing, second edition, is organized into five units. Each unit opens with a self-assessment section and closes with a self-evaluation section. The self-assessment and self-evaluation exercises are structured to help you identify cultural biases and prejudices, overcome communication barriers, and develop your own communication style.

Unit One: Exploring Transcultural Communication focuses on concepts that are the prerequisites for developing transcultural communication skills. This unit builds on the fundamental principle that all individuals have cultural traditions that influence their patterns of interaction and communication. The chapters in Unit One will help you recognize that your interactions with patients represent the values of your culture, the values of the nursing subculture, and your patients' culturally-influenced values and communication styles.

Specifically, the chapters in this unit discuss:

- The growing demand for transcultural communication in health care settings.
- Building blocks that form the basis for transcultural communication: culture, cultural values, beliefs, behavior, and communication.
- Stumbling blocks that impede transcultural communication: lack of knowledge, fear and distrust, racism, bias, ethnocentrism, stereotyping, ritualistic behavior, language barriers, and conflicting perceptions and expectations.
- Interactions between health care system subcultures that may positively or negatively affect transcultural communication; for example interactions between Western health care, hospital, nursing, and patient subcultures.

Unit Two: Developing Transcultural Communication Skills concentrates on helping you to develop your observational, listening, nonverbal, and verbal transcultural communication skills. Unit Two offers practical suggestions for developing relationships with patients from different cultures by conveying empathy, showing respect, building trust, establishing rapport, listening actively, and providing appropriate feedback. This unit gives specific directions in how to:

- Explore transcultural situations as a participant–observer by interacting with people from different cultures as they go about their normal lives; for example, exploring ethnic neighborhoods and attending family celebrations and religious ceremonies.
- Establish a therapeutic relationship and communication with patients from diverse cultures.
- Overcome transcultural communication barriers.
- Communicate with patients who are not proficient in English, with or without the help of a professional interpreter.
- Work successfully with professional medical interpreters.

Unit 3: Using Transcultural Communication to Elicit Assessment Data and Develop Nursing Diagnoses builds on the important premise that a thorough cultural assessment of the patient forms the basis for culturally-appropriate nursing diagnoses and interventions. One goal of transcultural communication is to decrease the imposition of Western health care values on patients when these values hinder patients from achieving their own health objectives. By carefully assessing patients and learning more about their perspective, you should be able to (1) decrease transcultural conflicts, (2) evaluate the patient's culturally influenced needs, (3) determine the patient's nursing diagnoses, and (4) arrive at a mutually agreeable plan of care.

Specifically, Unit Three should help you to:

- Develop the art of eliciting culturally-related information from patients.
- Ask questions that will elicit the patient's perspective on illness, as well as the viewpoints of the patient's family and support group.
- Formulate and write culturally-appropriate nursing diagnoses that are based on a culturally-competent nursing assessment.
- Inspire other health care professionals to use and promote culturally-appropriate nursing diagnoses.

Unit Four: Using Transcultural Communication to Plan and Implement Care moves from how to perform a cultural assessment to how to use transcultural communication for care planning, teaching patients, and providing care. This unit provides:

- Techniques for developing plans of care that are tailored to meet the patient's cultural perceptions and expectations.
- Techniques for assessing the learning needs of patients from other cultures.
- Techniques for teaching patients from other cultures about prescribed medications, procedures, hospital policies, life style changes that they may need to make, and home care following discharge.
- Techniques for assisting patients and families from other cultures cope with pain, grief, dying, and death.

You may wonder: "How can I possibly learn enough about all the different cultural groups to plan for, care for, and instruct my patients?" Remember that it is not necessary to know in detail the values and expected behaviors of different cultural groups. It **is** important to learn about each patient's cultural perception of illness and health care, as well as each patient's culturally determined expectations for care.

Unit Five: Transcultural Communication Skills Between Health Care Providers focuses on communication between health care providers in the health care workplace, which is often a multinational, multicultural setting.

This unit presents:

- Major barriers that impede transcultural communication between health care providers from different cultures; for example clashes in values and language differences.

- Different approaches you can use to improve your transcultural communication with physicians, other nurses, and ancillary personnel from different cultures.

- Techniques for the nurse manager who identifies conflicts among workers and tensions between nurses and patients.

SPECIAL FEATURES

Special features of this book include the following exercises, techniques, tests, boxes, and resources:

- **Self-assessment exercises** are at the beginning of each unit. These exercises are designed to increase self-awareness; identify underlying attitudes, biases, and prejudices that can block your transcultural communication; and assess your transcultural communication style.

- **Self-evaluation exercises** are at the end of every unit. These exercises will help to evaluate your progress as you proceed through the chapters in each unit.

- **Transcultural Communication Diary**, included in the self-assessment and self-evaluation exercises, will allow you to record, analyze, and cultivate the transcultural communication insights and skills you are learning about in each unit.

- **Key Terms** at the beginning of every chapter list the 8–10 concepts that are central to comprehending the chapter. You should understand the terms and their relevance to transcultural communication after completing each chapter.

- **Learning Objectives** at the beginning of each chapter will encourage you to focus on the key concepts, strategies, and approaches that are addressed in the chapter content.

- **Step-by-step transcultural communication techniques,** using real world scenarios, are located throughout the book. These techniques provide clear directions for improving your communication with patients and health care providers from other cultures.

- **Communication Considerations** boxes serve to highlight important information about transcultural communication.

- **Organizations and Agencies** that provide transcultural information and resources are located in Appendix I. These resources
  include professional organizations, government agencies, ethnic and
  minority organizations, international agencies, refugee centers, and
  telephone information lines.

- **Annotated lists of suggested books and films** with a transcultural theme are located in Appendix II. These books (fiction and non-
  fiction) and films demonstrate communication between cultures, and
  they have been selected to enhance your understanding of transcultural interaction.

CONTRIBUTORS

Lydia DeSantis, PhD, RN, FAAN
University of Miami
Coral Gables, Florida

Oneida M. Hughes, PhD, RN
Texas Woman's University
Dallas, Texas

Carol J. Leppa, PhD, RN
University of Washington
Seattle, Washington

Margaret A. McKenna, PhD, MN, MPH
University of Washington
Seattle, Washington

Linda Sue Smith, DSN, RN
Food and Drug Administration,
Special Government Employee
Washington, DC

REVIEWERS

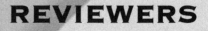

G. Rumay Alexander, MSN, EdD, RN, BSN
Director of Multicultural Affairs and
 The University of North Carolina at Chapel Hill
School of Nursing
Durham, North Carolina

Joan H. Baldwin, DNSc, MA, MSN, RN, BSN
Professor of Nursing
Brigham Young University
Provo, Utah

Dr. Merle Brown, PhD, APN Clinician
Online Nursing Faculty
University of Phoenix
Phoenix, Arizona
and
Essex County College of Nursing
Adjunct Faculty
Newark, New Jersey

Carmen Dombrovschi, MSN, RNC
Instructor of Nursing
Gateway Community College
Phoenix, Arizona

Lori Edwards, MPH, RN, BSN, CS
Instructor
Johns Hopkins University
School of Nursing
Baltimore, Maryland

Dr. Larry Purnell, PhD, RN, FAAN
Professor of Nursing
University of Delaware
Newark, Delaware

Catherine Sikorski, MSN, APRN, BC
Clinical Instructor of Nursing
Wayne State University
Detroit, Michigan

Laura Smith-McKenna, DNSc, RN
Assistant Professor of Nursing
Samuel Merritt College
Oakland, California

TECHNICAL REVIEWER

Dr. Barbara Jones Warren, PhD, APRN, BC
Professor of Nursing
The Ohio State University
Health Sciences Center
Columbus, Ohio

UNIT ONE

Exploring Transcultural Communication

UNIT ONE
ASSESSMENT

ASSESSING YOUR TRANSCULTURAL COMMUNICATION GOALS AND BASIC KNOWLEDGE

Exercise One: Assessing Your Personal Objectives

What is your objective for studying transcultural communication? Check the points listed below that apply to you or write down your own objectives.

My personal objectives are to:

_____ Learn about the effects of culture on communication.

_____ Identify my own patterns of communication that have been influenced by my culture.

_____ Develop skill in identifying patients' different cultural beliefs.

_____ Decrease the frustration I experience when working with patients whose primary language is not English.

_____ Improve my effectiveness in conveying information to patients from different cultures.

_____ Overcome cultural biases that are blocking my ability to relate well to patients from different cultural backgrounds.

_____ Sharpen my skills in assessing patients who speak little English and who have cultural values different from my own.

_____ Improve my ability to convey health information to patients from different cultures.

_____ Give more culturally sensitive care.

My other objectives for studying this book are to: _____

_____

_____

Exercise Two: Assessing How You Relate to Various Groups of People in Society

The following self-test questionnaire will help you assess how you relate to various groups of people in society. This assessment, in turn, will help you assess how you relate to various groups of patients in your care. Take a moment now to complete and score this test.

2

SELF-TEST QUESTIONNAIRE

How Do You Relate to Various Groups of People in Society?

Described below are different levels of response you might have toward a person.

Levels of Response:
1. *Greet:* I feel I can greet this person warmly and welcome him or her sincerely.
2. *Accept:* I feel I can honestly accept this person as he or she is and be comfortable enough to listen to his or her problems.
3. *Help:* I feel I would genuinely try to help this person with his or her problems as they might be related to or arise from the label or stereotype given to him or her.
4. *Background:* I feel I have the background of knowledge and experience to be able to help this person.
5. *Advocate:* I feel I could honestly be an advocate for this person.

The following is a list of individuals. Read down the list and place a checkmark by anyone you "would *not* greet or would hesitate to greet." Then move to response level 2, "accept," and follow the same procedure. Try to respond honestly, not as you think might be socially or professionally desirable. Your answers are only for your personal use in clarifying your initial reactions to different people.

Individual	1 Greet	2 Accept	3 Help	4 Background	5 Advocate
1. Haitian	☐	☐	☐	☐	☐
2. Child abuser	☐	☐	☐	☐	☐
3. Jew	☐	☐	☐	☐	☐
4. Iranian American	☐	☐	☐	☐	☐
5. Neo-Nazi	☐	☐	☐	☐	☐
6. Mexican American	☐	☐	☐	☐	☐
7. IV drug user	☐	☐	☐	☐	☐
8. Catholic	☐	☐	☐	☐	☐
9. Senile elderly person	☐	☐	☐	☐	☐
10. Teamster Union member	☐	☐	☐	☐	☐

(continues)

Individual	1 Greet	2 Accept	3 Help	4 Background	5 Advocate
11. Native American	☐	☐	☐	☐	☐
12. Prostitute	☐	☐	☐	☐	☐
13. Jehovah's Witness	☐	☐	☐	☐	☐
14. Cerebral palsied person	☐	☐	☐	☐	☐
15. E.R.A. proponent	☐	☐	☐	☐	☐
16. Vietnamese American	☐	☐	☐	☐	☐
17. Gay/Lesbian	☐	☐	☐	☐	☐
18. Muslim	☐	☐	☐	☐	☐
19. Person with AIDS	☐	☐	☐	☐	☐
20. Communist	☐	☐	☐	☐	☐
21. Black American	☐	☐	☐	☐	☐
22. Unmarried expectant teen	☐	☐	☐	☐	☐
23. Protestant	☐	☐	☐	☐	☐
24. Amputee	☐	☐	☐	☐	☐
25. Ku Klux Klansman	☐	☐	☐	☐	☐
26. White Anglo-Saxon	☐	☐	☐	☐	☐
27. Alcoholic	☐	☐	☐	☐	☐
28. Amish person	☐	☐	☐	☐	☐
29. Person with cancer	☐	☐	☐	☐	☐
30. Nuclear armament proponent	☐	☐	☐	☐	☐

Scoring Guide: The previous activity may help you anticipate difficulty in working with some clients at various levels. The thirty types of individuals can be grouped into five categories: ethnic/racial, social issues/problems, religious, physically/mentally challenged, and political. Transfer your checkmarks to the following form. A concentration of checks within a specific category of individuals or at specific levels may indicate a conflict that could hinder you from rendering effective professional help.

Individual	1 Greet	2 Accept	3 Help	4 Background	5 Advocate
Ethnic/Racial					
1. Haitian	☐	☐	☐	☐	☐
4. Iranian American	☐	☐	☐	☐	☐
6. Mexican American	☐	☐	☐	☐	☐
11. Native American	☐	☐	☐	☐	☐
16. Vietnamese American	☐	☐	☐	☐	☐
21. Black American	☐	☐	☐	☐	☐
26. White Anglo-Saxon	☐	☐	☐	☐	☐
Social Issues/Problems					
2. Child abuser	☐	☐	☐	☐	☐
7. IV drug user	☐	☐	☐	☐	☐
12. Prostitute	☐	☐	☐	☐	☐
17. Gay/Lesbian	☐	☐	☐	☐	☐
22. Unmarried expectant teen	☐	☐	☐	☐	☐
27. Alcoholic	☐	☐	☐	☐	☐
Religious					
3. Jew	☐	☐	☐	☐	☐
8. Catholic	☐	☐	☐	☐	☐
13. Jehovah's Witness	☐	☐	☐	☐	☐
18. Muslim	☐	☐	☐	☐	☐
23. Protestant	☐	☐	☐	☐	☐
28. Amish person	☐	☐	☐	☐	☐

(continues)

Individual	1 Greet	2 Accept	3 Help	4 Background	5 Advocate
Physically/Mentally challenged					
9. Senile elderly person	☐	☐	☐	☐	☐
14. Cerebral palsied person	☐	☐	☐	☐	☐
19. Person with AIDS	☐	☐	☐	☐	☐
24. Amputee	☐	☐	☐	☐	☐
29. Person with cancer	☐	☐	☐	☐	☐
Political					
5. Neo-Nazi	☐	☐	☐	☐	☐
10. Teamster Union member	☐	☐	☐	☐	☐
15. E.R.A. proponent	☐	☐	☐	☐	☐
20. Communist	☐	☐	☐	☐	☐
25. Ku Klux Klansman	☐	☐	☐	☐	☐
30. Nuclear armament proponent	☐	☐	☐	☐	☐

Reprinted by permission from Association for the Care of Children's Health (ACCH) 7910 Woodmont Ave. 300, Bethesda, MD, 20814, from *Strategies for working with culturally diverse communities and clients*, 1989, by E. Randall-David.

Exercise Three: Assessing Your Personal Responses to Transcultural Nursing Situations

When you are asked to care for a patient from a different cultural background, it is natural to have some concerns. How do you feel about working with patients who are from a culture very different from your own or who do not speak English? Are you worried that you will not be able to communicate clearly with these patients? Try to respond as honestly as possible to the statements below.

	Agree	Neutral	Disagree
People are the same. I don't behave any differently toward people from a cultural background that differs from mine.	_____	_____	_____
I always know what to say to someone from a different cultural background.	_____	_____	_____
I look forward to caring for a patient from a different cultural background.	_____	_____	_____
I know how to care for a patient who does not speak any English.	_____	_____	_____
I can learn something when I care for patients from diverse cultural backgrounds.	_____	_____	_____
I always introduce myself to the patient's family.	_____	_____	_____
I prefer to care for a patient from my own cultural group who speaks my language because it is easier.	_____	_____	_____

Exercise Four: Examining Your Cultural Values

This exercise is designed to help you explore your cultural values (which are most likely Western) in relationship to the cultural values of non-Western cultural groups. This exercise contains nine pairs of statements that have relevance to nursing. The statements on the left represent Western values; the statements on the right represent values held elsewhere in the world. As you rate each statement, *try to be as truthful with yourself as possible*. If you are really honest, you may be surprised at how many of your answers are heavily biased toward Western values.

CULTURAL VALUES

Directions

Circle 1 if you strongly agree with the statement on the left.
Circle 2 if you agree with the statement on the left.
Circle 3 if you agree with the statement on the right.
Circle 4 if you strongly agree with the statement on the right.

1. Responsible adults prepare for the future and strive to influence events in their lives.	1 2 3 4	Life follows a preordained course. The outcome of events is beyond our control.
2. It is confusing and dishonest to give vague and tentative answers.	1 2 3 4	It is best to avoid direct and honest answers because you may offend and embarrass others.
3. Intelligent, efficient people use their time well and are always punctual.	1 2 3 4	Being punctual to work or a meeting is not as important as enjoying relaxed and pleasant times with family and friends.
4. Stoicism is the appropriate response to severe pain.	1 2 3 4	Loudly crying out and moaning are appropriate responses to severe pain.
5. It is not wise to accept a gift from a person you do not know.	1 2 3 4	It is important to accept gifts and thus avoid insulting the giver.
6. It is a sign of friendliness to address people by their first name.	1 2 3 4	It is disrespectful to address people by their first name unless they give you permission to do so.
7. The best way to gain information is to ask direct questions.	1 2 3 4	It is rude and intrusive to obtain information by asking direct questions.
8. Direct eye contact shows that you are an honest person and that you are interested in the other person.	1 2 3 4	Avoiding direct eye contact is acceptable and may communicate respect especially with elders and those in positions of authority.
9. Ultimately, the needs of the individual are more important than the needs of the family.	1 2 3 4	The needs of the family far outweigh the needs of the individual.

Adapted from Renwick, G. W., & Rhinesmith, S. H. *An exercise in cultural analysis for managers.* Chicago: Intercultural Press, Inc. Published in: Thiederman, S.B. Ethnocentrism: A barrier to effective health care. *Nurse Practitioner, 11*(8), 52–59, 1986.

Exercise Five: Setting Up Your *Transcultural Interaction Diary*

Perhaps at some time you have kept a diary or a journal for recording your thoughts, feelings, activities, and memorable events. To improve your transcultural communication, you need to set up and keep a *Transcultural Interaction Diary*. This diary will provide you with a record of your experiences with patients and other health care professionals from different cultures. You can use your diary to (1) record your transcultural verbal and nonverbal communications, (2) analyze your feelings concerning these transactions, (3) plan strategies for improving your transcultural communications, and (4) record the outcomes from these strategies.

To set up your *Transcultural Interaction Diary*, follow these simple steps:

1. Decide on a "form" for your diary. For example, you can use a legal pad, a spiral notebook, note cards, a "locked" diary, a book with blank pages, or computer disks.

2. Keep your diary in a private place. You will not feel as free to write about negative interactions or feelings if you think other people will read your material.

3. Write in your diary on a regular basis—preferably every time that you have a significant (very positive or negative) transcultural interaction. It is important to record conversations, thoughts, and feelings while they are still fresh in your memory.

4. Start to write in your diary *now*, before reading the chapters in this unit. Think back and record any significant transcultural interactions that you had before you entered nursing and since you have been in nursing. Be sure to write down both verbal and nonverbal communications, as well as the thoughts and feelings that you had during and after each interaction.

5. As you study Unit One, write down any *new* transcultural interactions in your diary. Note how you are using the information in each chapter to increase your ability to communicate with the different cultural groups within your health care subculture.

CHAPTER 1

Introduction to Transcultural Communication in Nursing

KEY TERMS

- Body Language
- Communication Competence
- Cultural Diversity
- Culturally Competent Care
- Dyad
- Exchange Process
- Oral Language
- Population Categories

OBJECTIVES

After completing this chapter, you should be able to:

- Begin to interact with your patients in an exchange–negotiation process.
- Describe the dimensions of communication competence.
- List and explain the six reasons transcultural communication is urgently needed in the health care workplace today.
- Discuss the danger of relying on the statistical categories developed by the U.S. government for categorizing people into five population groups.

INTRODUCTION

The delivery of health care depends on clear communication between the individuals who are involved—for example, patients, physicians, nurses, interpreters, and family members. Clear communication is essential in any health care context, be it a provider's office, an acute care unit, a patient's home, or an extended care facility.

The most common form of communication is the **dyad**, or interaction between two people. The dyad of a nurse and a patient is the primary form of nurse–patient interaction in most health care settings. Nurses may also speak to groups of people, and they may teach patients with similar needs in a classroom setting. An example is a prenatal class. But most often, the nurse communicates with one patient at a time, with the goal of making that exchange as effective, appropriate, and acceptable to both parties as possible.

Unfortunately, any communication between nurse and patient can be reduced in quality and marked by frustration. Frustration arises when the nurse gives too little attention to the cultural background of the patient and its influence on communication. This text focuses on how to improve the quality of transcultural communication between patients and nurses and between nurses and other staff members. To improve your interactions with people from diverse backgrounds, you will need to learn more about different cultures and develop your communication skills.

COMMUNICATION: A CORNERSTONE FOR NURSING PRACTICE

To successfully work with patients from other cultures, you must continually strive for clear communication and mutual understanding. In many interactions, communication is cloudy because nurses incorrectly assume that their patients understand what they are trying to communicate.

> **• • • • COMMUNICATION CONSIDERATIONS • • • •**
>
> To improve your interaction with patients from other cultures, you should assess each patient's level of understanding rather than assume that a patient understands what you are saying.

One way to improve transcultural communication effectiveness is to think of your interaction with a patient as an **exchange process**, not as a one-sided provider-to-patient path of information. A satisfactory health care interaction between a provider and a patient is really one of exchange and negotiation.

Consider this exchange process as a scale that can be weighted in favor of one side or that can be balanced between your proposed plan of care and your patient's beliefs and preferences for care. For example, your patient may believe strongly in complementary (alternative) therapies. If that is the case, you could ignore the patient's interest in complementary therapies, a strategy that would probably upset the patient. Or you could take the patient's beliefs into consideration as you develop your care plan.

In an exchange with a patient from another culture, you need to know:

1. How and when to start a conversation.
2. How best to be understood; for example, you may need an interpreter.
3. How to respond to a patient's gestures or questions.
4. How to be sensitive to the patient's reactions.
5. How to listen to the patient's concerns.
6. How to take the patient's illness and health-related beliefs into consideration as you plan care.

These dimensions are the basis for **communication competence**. The primary objective of this textbook is to bring you closer to transcultural communication competence. To improve your transcultural communication skills, read each chapter carefully and work through the self-assessment and self-evaluation exercises that are at the beginning and end of each unit. You can also develop competence in transcultural communication by following these steps:

- Assess your own cultural background.
- Identify the values that underlie your behavior.
- Recognize that communication is influenced and determined by your culture.
- Recognize that there are many cultures that interact in a health care setting.

LANGUAGE AND COMMUNICATION

Language is the primary means used by humans to communicate with each other. Humans have developed written, sign, and oral languages in order to share messages. Humans use language to express ideas, feelings, and emotions; to communicate information, reactions, and directions to each other; and to negotiate with each other.

Oral language is a feature of every society. In a health care setting, oral language is used to verbally communicate with patients and other health care professionals. Nurses need to recognize that individuals also communicate in nonverbal ways.

People communicate nonverbally with **body language**, a topic that is discussed in greater detail in Chapter 4. Sign language, a form of body language, is the native language of members of deaf communities. It is important to remember that there are many cross-cultural similarities in body language, but there are also key differences. The meaning of different gestures varies from culture to culture. Never assume that a gesture holds the same meaning for you and your patient—especially if your patient is from another culture.

As you work with patients, you will encounter a great diversity in spoken languages. For instance, over 6000 languages and dialects are spoken today. Mandarin Chinese is spoken by approximately 836 million people. In the late 1990s, there were nearly as many Spanish speakers (who number 332 million) as there are Hindi speakers (who number 333 million worldwide) (Microsoft, 1996). There are 322 million English speakers. If we include individuals who speak English as a second language, with approximately 418 million speakers, then English is the second most widely spoken language (with Mandarin Chinese being the most widely spoken).

Although you cannot expect to be familiar with even a portion of these languages, you can still find ways to communicate with patients who do not speak or understand English. In Chapter 10, you will find helpful suggestions on how to communicate clearly with patients who are not proficient in English, with or without an interpreter.

THE GROWING DEMAND FOR TRANSCULTURAL COMMUNICATION

There are mounting reasons for nurses and health care providers to become competent in transcultural communication. The motivating forces that provide the momentum for implementing transcultural communication come from several sources:

1. There is increasing ethnic, racial, and **cultural diversity** in the composition of the U.S. population.

2. Patients represent many cultural, ethnic, and disenfranchised populations, and they have different culturally influenced patterns of behavior and expectations for care. Moreover, patients are increasingly more diverse in heritage, experiences, and lifestyle.

3. *Cultural meanings in health care:* The meaning of health and illness varies from group to group. An understanding of various meanings and cultural significance of health and illness, as well as traditional practices, is essential for planning interventions that are culturally sensitive. Health does not only refer to one's state of being. It is connected to how individuals perceive and construct reality, and reality is based on cultural experiences, beliefs, values, and practices.

4. *Behavioral responses to health care services:* The way patients and families respond to services they receive is influenced by various cultural factors, including their belief system and world view. For example, if a patient explains illness as caused by supernatural or religious forces, the patient's response to treatment will be positive if some type of spiritual/religious intervention is included in the treatment plan. Level of adherence to treatment and compliance is influenced by the cultural beliefs and practices of the patient.

5. The meaning of health and illness varies from group to group.

6. Patients' behavioral responses to health care services are influenced by their cultural background.

7. Settings for health care delivery are multicultural and multinational.

8. The nursing profession has a commitment to provide humanistic, culturally appropriate care.

Increasing Diversity in Population Composition

The ethnic and racial composition of the population of the United States has changed dramatically since the 1990s as reported in Census 2000, which shows a racially diverse United States (U.S. Census Bureau, 2001). There is increasing diversity in languages, beliefs, lifestyles, and practices among residents in rural and urban areas throughout the country. The percentage of the U.S. population that is white has decreased since the 1970s. This reduction in percentage is due in part to increasing immigration from Asian and Latin American nations and in part to a higher population growth rate among blacks.

Making a direct comparison between data from the 1990 census or an earlier census is difficult and complex because the question on race was changed for Census 2000. In Census 2000, respondents were asked to report one or more races in which they consider themselves to belong, a question that had not been asked in earlier censuses. As a result, the data collected for Census 2000 fall into two groups: (1) persons who reported belonging to one race only and (2) persons who reported belonging to more than one race.

Census 2000 showed that the U.S. population was 281,421,906 people, with 75.1% white, 12.3% black, 3.8% Asian, 12.5% Hispanic, and 1% Native American. It is projected that by the year 2020 the population will reach 323 million; 60% of this increase will be due to more births than deaths and 40% to immigration (Spector, 2004).

Because of this increase in the population of ethnic groups, health care services will have to address the needs of patients from diverse cultural, ethnic, and racial backgrounds.

Multicultural Patient Groups

It is not unusual to hear a number of languages and dialects spoken among patients in a large medical center, especially in an urban or suburban setting. In a northwestern city in the United States, each of the hospitals, clinics, and other health care settings may care for families who speak as many as 40 different languages.

Nurses will continue to encounter patients in many different health care settings who speak a language other than English. According to the U.S. Census Bureau (2001), in 1990 more than 32 million Americans spoke a language other than English at home. By the year 2000, that number had increased to almost 46 million. More than 28 million Americans speak Spanish, and almost 7 million speak an Asian or a Pacific Islander language at home.

Multinational and Multicultural Workplaces

Nurses and other health care providers practice in a multicultural environment, even if they think of themselves as belonging to one culture or as "just being American." The misunderstandings that develop in health care settings may occur between providers, as well as between patients and providers, from different cultural backgrounds. Many nurses would find these words familiar: "I can't understand why this family won't do what I ask," or "I hope I don't have to work with that nurse again. I'm never sure he understands what I am talking about."

Two goals of this book are to (1) discuss the barriers that can block transcultural communication between nurses and other health care providers and (2) provide clear guidelines for recognizing and overcoming these barriers in the workplace.

• • • COMMUNICATION CONSIDERATIONS • • •

To work effectively as team members and provide safe patient care, nurses must commit to improving communication in the workplace, particularly when team members are from diverse cultures.

Professional Mandate for Culturally Competent Care

The National League for Nursing and many state boards of nursing have acknowledged that cultural considerations are an important aspect of patient care. Furthermore, these organizations have made a commitment to include cultural concepts (including transcultural communication) in the educational preparation of nurses (Andrews & Boyle, 2002). The American Academy of Nursing has also pledged to (1) promote the development and maintenance of a disciplinary knowledge base in transcultural nursing and (2) foster nursing expertise in **culturally competent care**. Culturally competent care is defined by the American Academy of Nursing (1992) as a complex integration of knowledge, attitudes, and skills that enhance cross-cultural communication and appropriate and effective interactions. Cultural competence also has been defined as a process that includes components of cultural awareness, cultural knowledge, cultural skills, cultural encounters, and cultural desire (Campinha-Bacote & Muñoz, 2001).

In addition, all nurses need to commit themselves to enhancing their knowledge of different cultures and developing their skills in transcultural communication. You can gain a knowledge of different cultures by reading about cultures, seeing films about different cultures, talking with patients or co-workers about their cultural backgrounds, or acting as a participant-observer in a cultural setting such as an ethnic neighborhood. You can develop transcultural communication skills by first assessing your level of skill, practicing various techniques to improve your skills, evaluating your new skills, and deciding what improvements you still need to make.

• • • COMMUNICATION CONSIDERATIONS • • •

Improving your transcultural communication with patients and team members is an ongoing process. Every new person you meet who is from another culture will help to broaden your appreciation of different cultures and improve your transcultural communication skills.

VITAL REMARKS AND SPECIAL CAUTIONS

For the purpose of collecting statistics, the U.S. and Canadian governments have categorized people into five general **population categories**: white, black, Hispanic, Asian, and Native American. These categories are used in health care settings as well as in schools, government facilities, and businesses. Unfortunately, the use of these five categories has tended to diminish the very essence of quality health care. That is, the widespread use of such broad categories has blurred or even extinguished the crucial cultural differences between the individuals and the groups within each population census category (Andrews & Boyle, 2002).

> ### • • • • COMMUNICATION CONSIDERATIONS • • • •
>
> People should not be stereotyped simply because they are members of a broad, statistically defined, racial or ethnic category. Although patients and health care providers may share values with other people from their race or culture, they are first and foremost individuals.

It is important to recognize that within each of the broad, statistical categories there are numerous cultural groups. These groups are characterized by variations in lifestyle, values and beliefs, health- and illness-related practices, preferences for care, and family member patterns of interaction. For example, many cultural groups are included in the category of *white* (sometimes also referred to as Anglo-American or Caucasian). Individuals in these groups may trace their heritage to a European nation, Australia, North America, or many other nations and regions. Among individuals who are white, the largest group of 58 million people have a German ancestry. Another 39 million Americans trace their roots to Ireland, and more than 32.6 million Americans have an English ancestry (U.S. Census Bureau, 2001).

There is also great diversity among the individuals who are included in the *Hispanic* population category. There are differences in their countries of origin, in the dialects spoken, and in customs and beliefs, including practices related to health and illness. For example, among Spanish speakers, there are many variations in the use of words and expressions. Patients from different states in Mexico have different dialects, and they do not necessarily understand individuals from Puerto Rico or Cuba. Recent immigrants from Mexico may speak an Indian dialect or a mixture of Spanish and Mixtec.

The term *black* is similarly very inclusive and may refer to individuals who are recent refugees or immigrants from African nations or individuals who can trace their heritage through multiple generations of residence in the United States. Furthermore, the term *Native American* too often blurs the distinctions among members of more than 500 Native American nations who reside in North America. Likewise, the term *Asian* refers to the Japanese, Chinese, Indochinese, Filipino, Korean, Vietnamese, and Indian populations, each of which contains numerous, diverse subcultures.

In this book, the five population census categories are presented. However, we emphasize that each of these categories contains many different cultural groups, which, in turn, are composed of people with their own individual ideas, beliefs, and values. Each chapter contains examples and brief clinical interactions that illustrate how to use transcultural communication skills to interact with patients from a variety of cultural backgrounds. Chapter 15 also describes skills for interacting with staff members from diverse backgrounds.

COMMUNICATION CONSIDERATIONS

Always consider patients and co-workers from other cultures as individuals with unique experiences and expectations, and then as members of different cultures.

REFERENCES

American Academy of Nursing. (1992). AAN expert panel report: Culturally competent health care. *Nursing Outlook, 40*(6), 277–283.

Andrews, M. M., & Boyle, J. S. (2002). *Transcultural concepts in nursing care* (4th ed.). Philadelphia: Lippincott.

Campinha-Bacote, J., & Muñoz, C. (2001). A guiding framework for delivering culturally competent services in case management. *The Case Manager, 12*, 48–52.

Spector, R. E. (2004). *Cultural diversity in health and illness* (6th ed.). Upper Saddle River, NJ: Pearson Prentice Hall.

U.S. Census Bureau. (2001). *U.S. Department of Commerce News.* Washington DC. Retrieved March 12, 2001. From: *www.census.gov/PressRelease2001.*

SUGGESTED READINGS

American Demographics Inc. (1991). American diversity: What the 1990 Census reveals about population growth, blacks, Hispanics, Asians, ethnic diversity, and children—and what it means to you. *American Demographics Desk Reference Series*. No 1.

Lester, N. (1998). Cultural competence: A nursing dialogue. *American Journal of Nursing, 98*(8), 26–34.

Lester, N. (1998). Cultural competence: A nursing dialogue. (Part II). *American Journal of Nursing, 98*(9), 36–44.

Microsoft. (1996). *Microsoft Encarta 97 Encyclopedia*. Microsoft Corporation.

CHAPTER 2

Transcultural Communication Building Blocks: Culture and Cultural Values

KEY TERMS

- African American
- Amor Propio
- Ashkenazi Jew
- Asian
- Black
- Conservative Jew
- Cultural Values
- Culture
- Culture Shock
- Deitsch
- Demut
- Filipino
- Galang
- Gelassenheit
- Hasidic Jew
- Hispanic
- Holocaust
- Kosher
- Lace Curtain Irish

- Latino
- Monotheistic
- Muslim
- Native American
- Old Order Amish
- Orthodox Jew
- Pilipino
- Pogrom
- Reform Jew
- Sabra
- Sephardic Jew
- Shanty Irish
- Subculture
- Tagalog
- Torah
- Treyf
- Tzedakah
- WASP
- Zerangi

OBJECTIVES

After completing this chapter, you should be able to:

- Define *culture* and discuss its role in determining the philosophy and values of individuals and groups.
- Define *subculture* and describe the different subcultures that are a part of American culture.
- Define *cultural values* and provide at least seven reasons that values are so important.
- Differentiate between the major value systems of different cultural groups.
- Acquire information about the beliefs and values of the specific cultural groups with whom you routinely work.

INTRODUCTION

Transcultural communication involves the successful interchange of ideas and feelings between people from different cultures. For nurses, the ability to communicate transculturally with patients and their families often spells the difference between success and frustration when assessing patients and providing their care. The study of culture provides the foundation necessary for understanding and fostering transcultural communication. This chapter discusses the meaning of culture and explores the ways in which culture affects a person's values, beliefs, behavior, and communication style.

CULTURE

Culture refers to the common lifestyles, languages, behavior patterns, traditions, and beliefs that are learned and passed from one generation to the next. Culture helps to determine a person's world view, or philosophy of life, and it influences how each of us views our relationship to our surrounding environment, religion, time, and each other. Culture provides each person with specific rules for dealing with the universal events of life—birth, mating, childrearing, illness, pain, and death.

Although culture provides strength and stability, it is never static. Cultural groups face continual challenges from such powerful forces as environmental upheavals, plagues, wars, migrations, the influx of immigrants, and the growth of new technologies. As a result, cultures change and evolve over time.

Culture is learned and then shared. People learn about their culture from parents, teachers, religious and political leaders, and respected peers. As children grow up, they gradually internalize the values and beliefs of their culture, and they, in turn, share these values and beliefs with their children.

Normally, children learn about their culture while growing up. However, when people emigrate from their native culture into a new culture, they often experience **culture shock**. Culture shock develops when the values and beliefs upheld by this new culture are radically different from those of the person's native culture. For successful assimilation into a new culture, immigrants must learn and internalize that culture's important values.

In addition to belonging to a major cultural group, people also belong to a variety of **subcultures**, or smaller groups within a culture. Each subculture has its own value system and related expectations for behavior. Subcultures may be based on:

1. Professional and occupational affiliations (registered nurses).
2. Nationality or race (a shared historical and political past).
3. Age groups (adolescents, senior citizens).
4. Gender (feminists, mens' groups).
5. Socioeconomic factors (the working class, the middle class, the upper class).
6. Political viewpoints (Democrat, Republican).
7. Sexual orientation (gay and lesbian groups).

For example, when you studied to be a nurse, you entered a subculture, and initially you probably suffered from some degree of culture shock. You had to learn a whole new value system. During your years of study, you gradually internalized the values taught by your instructors. Eventually, you became comfortable with the values and behaviors you learned in your school of nursing, and, by the time you graduated, you had been assimilated into the professional nursing subculture.

Upon admission to a hospital, patients also become members of a subculture. In this world filled with strange sights, unfamiliar sounds, and strangers, many patients experience culture shock. This shock intensifies for patients who are recent immigrants or who do not speak English.

• • • COMMUNICATION CONSIDERATIONS • • •

Because nurses and patients belong to different subcultures, their interaction is always to some extent transcultural, even when the nurse and patient come from the same general culture.

In summary, culture has a powerful impact on individuals, groups, and entire societies, influencing all aspects of human life. Cultures and subcultures provide strategies and methods for coping with life's ever-changing challenges and demands. Family, childrearing, economics, education, health beliefs, and health care are all dramatically influenced by culture and the values and beliefs that it engenders.

CULTURAL VALUES

Cultural values are principles or standards that members of a cultural group share in common. Values dramatically differ from culture to culture. People educated in mainstream, white, American, middle-class culture may have very different values from people raised in the many and varied Asian, Hispanic, black, or Native American cultures. Accepting and respecting the values of patients from other cultures is the first step toward successful transcultural communication.

Values serve several important functions:

1. They provide people with a set of rules by which to govern their lives.

2. They serve as a basis for attitudes, beliefs, and behaviors.

3. They help to guide actions and decisions.

4. They give direction to people's lives and help them solve common problems.

5. They influence how individuals perceive and react to other individuals.

6. They help determine basic attitudes regarding personal, social, and philosophical issues.

7. They reflect a person's identity and provide a basis for self-evaluation.

VALUES OF MAJOR AMERICAN CULTURAL GROUPS

The following general guidelines compare and contrast the basic traditional values of the five major cultural groups that are predominant in American society: white, Asian/Pacific Islanders, Hispanic, black, and Native American. However, it is vital to recognize that many individuals do not follow their culture's traditional values either because they have assimilated the values of a different culture or because they have formulated their own value system. Although these guidelines will help you understand a patient's general cultural background, some of your patients may believe in values that are different from those traditionally accepted in their cultures.

••• COMMUNICATION CONSIDERATIONS •••

Remember that each person is first and foremost an individual, and secondly a member of a cultural group.

Mainstream White American Values

White European Americans have diverse backgrounds with multicultural origins. Most of these groups emigrated to the United States between 1820 and 1990 from countries such as Germany, Italy, the United Kingdom, Hungary, and the countries of the former Soviet Union. Even as the United States moves toward diversity, the white population remains the majority group, constituting 75.1% of the population in the year 2000 (Spector, 2004). It is therefore important to understand the health values and practices of this group.

The prevailing value system for many mainstream white Americans is primarily based on the white, Anglo-Saxon, Protestant (**WASP**) ethic (Sue & Sue, 1990). This ethic traces its origins to the white Protestants who came to this country from Northern Europe over two centuries ago. Values that still dominate the white American middle-class ethic include independence, individuality, wealth, comfort, cleanliness, achievement, punctuality, hard work, aggression, assertiveness, rationality, an orientation toward the future, and mastery of one's own fate (Andrews & Boyle, 2002; Edmission, 1997).

Traditionally, most white Americans have wanted to be recognized as *individuals* rather than as members of groups. Thus white Americans, unlike members of many other cultures, tend to be competitive with each other rather than cooperative. Mainstream American culture also values the nuclear family and its traditions.

••• COMMUNICATION CONSIDERATIONS •••

Many white Americans do not belong to the mainstream culture, but instead belong to ethnic subcultures that hold strong values of their own (e.g., Irish, Jewish, Iranian, German, Italian, Norwegian, Appalachian, and Amish subcultures).

Asian/Pacific Islander Values

Within the United States, **Asian** (or *Asian American*) is a term that primarily encompasses the Japanese, Chinese, Filipino, Korean, Vietnamese, Cambodian, Laotian, Thai, Indonesian, Pakistani, Hmong, and Indian populations. These populations are highly diverse; indeed, members of these groups speak different languages and encounter different life experiences. The Asian-American population is growing rapidly. The 1990 census estimated the annual rate of growth of the Asian-American population to be 4%. In 2000, there were 11.9 million Asians within the United States, and that population may increase significantly more by the year 2010 (U.S. Census Bureau, 2001a).

Traditional Asian values are firmly rooted in traditional religious beliefs. Chinese, Vietnamese, and Korean values have been greatly influenced by Buddhism, Taoism, Christianity, and Confucianism (Compton's, 1995).

- *Buddhism* is a doctrine that is attributed to Siddhartha Gautama, the *Buddha* or *The Enlightened One*. Buddha lived around 2500 years ago in India. Buddhism teaches that suffering is an inevitable part of life. Devout Buddhists believe that by extinguishing their sense of self and their desires, they can pass beyond suffering into a state of perfect illumination or enlightenment, called Nirvana. One-eighth of the world's population believes in Buddhism.

- *Taoism*, another Eastern philosophy and religion, is based on the teachings of Lao-tse who lived in China during the sixth century BC. The word *Tao* means "way," suggesting a way of thinking and living. As is the God of the Christians and Jews, Tao is viewed as the essential unifying element of all that is. Taoism teaches that a person should cultivate a mystical relationship to the Tao, shun worldly desires, and avoid lusting after wealth and power. For a Taoist, the most important goal is to live an orderly life that is in harmony with the universe.

- *Christianity* is based on the teachings of Jesus of Nazareth, who was born in Bethlehem of Judea more than 2000 years ago. More than 1 billion people throughout the world believe in the teachings of Jesus Christ. Christianity is split into many different groups, the three largest being the Roman Catholic church, Eastern Orthodox churches, and Protestant churches. Although different churches have their own interpretation of Christian doctrine, all churches agree that the ideal Christian is compassionate, kind, humble, gentle, patient, and forgiving.

- *Confucianism* was founded by the great teacher Confucius, who lived from 551 to 479 BC. Because of his teachings and wise sayings (which are similar to the proverbs in the Bible), Confucius was revered in China almost like a god. Temples erected to honor Confucius were built in most of the major cities in China. Although Confucianism is considered a religion, it is actually a moral code of conduct. Confucius encouraged his followers to live a virtuous life filled with goodness and kind deeds. Confucius also taught that it was important to be accountable to one's family and neighbors and that elders and well-educated people deserve special consideration and respect.

Japanese religious values are primarily based on Zen Buddhism and Shintoism, whereas the religious beliefs of East Indians evolved from Hinduism.

- *Zen Buddhism* is a form of Buddhism that was transplanted from China to Japan around the twelfth century AD. *Zen* is a Japanese term meaning "meditation." Zen Buddhism was the religion of the Samurai warriors during the fourteenth and fifteenth centuries, and it dominated Japanese culture during the sixteenth century. In the 1950s, Alan Watts, a British philosopher, introduced Americans to Zen Buddhism through his book *The Way of Zen.* Zen Buddhism teaches that there is only one reality and that this reality can be understood only through meditation and intuition, not through reason and analysis. Devout followers of Zen may seek to enter a monastery, where they and their masters can find enlightenment through a life devoted to service, prayer, and meditation (Compton's, 1995).

- *Shintoism, way of the gods* or *kami way*, is the indigenous religion of Japan. Ancient Shintoism arose from a belief in *kami*, which means "god" or "gods," "above," "superior," or "divine." Shintoists believe that because kami manifests itself in nature (mountains, trees, birds, rivers, and stars) and in human beings, the entire universe is bound together by kami. Today there are over 80,000 Shinto shrines throughout the world. As did their ancient predecessors, modern Shintoists strive to embrace kami in their daily lives by performing various rituals and by participating in Shinto festivals and holidays. Present-day Shintoists may also petition their deities for material blessings such as a new car or home (Zehavi, 1973; Zich, 1991).

- *Hinduism* is the major religion of the Indian subcontinent. The word *Hindu* is derived from an ancient Sanskrit term and means "dwellers by the Indus River." The dwellers are the people who developed the Indus Valley Civilization almost 4000 years ago. Hinduism has no founder and no specific doctrine. Whereas Hinduism is characterized by a great diversity of beliefs, most Hindus adhere to the following religious tenets:

1. There is only one God, called Brahman.

2. All forms of nature and life are sacred.

3. Individuals pass through many cycles of life and death (transmigration of souls), and they may be reincarnated as human beings, animals, or even plants.

4. The priesthood is hereditary, and individuals may become priests only through reincarnation.

5. The way an individual lives in this life determines the next life (the doctrine of karma, or law of cause and effect).

Today, 90% of Hindus live in India, and the remaining 10% dwell in South Africa, Trinidad, Europe, and the United States (Compton's, 1995; Miller & Goodin, 1995).

Traditional Asian values and mainstream American values may differ in several ways. Whereas Western culture values independence and self-reliance, many Asian cultures place a higher value on subordination of personal interests to those of the family. For instance, some Asian family members will likely put aside their own work, needs, and interests to care for a sick or elderly relative. Also, Asians usually have a strong group orientation, which extends to the workplace.

Example: Some Asian nurses may accept assignments without complaint that mainstream American nurses might resent. They do not complain because Asian nurses are more likely to value the *combined work* of the nursing team over the work of an individual nurse. In addition, an Asian nurse may feel that it is inappropriate for a subordinate to challenge a supervisor. American nurses who feel unfairly treated are more likely to complain to their supervisors than are Asian nurses.

Table 2-1 identifies traditional Asian values and representative mainstream American values. Remember, however, that individuals may hold some traditional Asian values and some mainstream American values. For example, a person might value older people and the past but also value young people and the future, a situation that could create a conflict when values clash. Another person's values may lie somewhere between traditional Asian and mainstream American values.

◆◆◆◆ **TABLE 2-1** ◆◆◆◆

Examples of Traditional Asian Values and Mainstream American Values

Asian Values	American Values
Group orientation	Independence, self-reliance, and individualism
Submission to authority	Resistance to authority
Extended family	Nuclear/blended family
Tradition	Innovation
Respect for elders	Emphasis on youth
Respect for the past	Future orientation
Conformity	Competition

Hispanic Values

Hispanic is a broad term that refers to:

   1. Groups with cultural and national identities arising from the Caribbean, Mexico, and Central and South America.

   2. Individuals who trace their ancestry to Spain and identify themselves as Hispanic.

Thus, the term *Hispanic* is not linked to race but rather to culture and nationality. The term *Hispanic* is generally preferred to *Chicano*. The word **Latino** is sometimes used as an alternative to *Hispanic*. Many people prefer *Latino* because it implies cultural ties to South America rather than to Spain (Barnhart & Metcalf, 1999). According to the 2000 census, in 2000, there were 35.3 million people of Hispanic origin in the United States, about 13% of the total population (U.S. Census Bureau, 2001b). In addition, the Census Bureau reports that by 2005, Hispanics will be the nation's largest minority group, outnumbering blacks, who are currently the leading minority (Holmes, 1998).

The Hispanics—including Mexican Americans, Cubans, Salvadorans, Guatemalans, Puerto Ricans, and others—greatly value the family and often place the needs of family members above the needs of individuals. Family members are typically respectful and affectionate toward one another. The extended family may include not only blood relatives but also nonblood relatives such as godparents.

Many Hispanics value the development and nurturing of close interpersonal relationships. When a Hispanic family member is ill, family members usually give their sick relative abundant physical and emotional support. Because family ties are so valued, Hispanic patients usually want extended family members present during a hospitalization. Also, some Hispanic family members prefer to be involved in the decisions pertaining to their loved one's care.

In addition to valuing the family, many Hispanics have traditionally valued religion, especially Catholicism and the celebration of the Catholic Mass. Because of a deep religious faith, many Hispanics believe in self-sacrifice, giving rather than taking, enduring hardships, and accepting fate. Finally, Hispanics typically value the present over the future. Although most Hispanics must work, many feel that it is equally important to take time to enjoy leisure activities with family members.

Table 2-2 summarizes some common differences in values between Hispanic culture and mainstream American culture. Remember, individuals may not subscribe to every value held by a group. Some individuals may hold both traditional Hispanic values and mainstream American values. A person's values can also be influenced by occupation, level of education, income and work status, as well as the values of family or significant others.

Black Values

The term **black**, as do the terms *Hispanic* and *Asian*, erroneously lumps together a highly diverse group of people who came to the United States from many parts of the world. According to the 2000 census, blacks are currently the largest minority group in the United States, constituting 12.3% of the total population (U.S. Census Bureau, 2001c). The black population is

◆◆◆◆ **TABLE 2-2** ◆◆◆◆

Examples of Traditional Hispanic Values and Mainstream American Values

Hispanic Values	American Values
Group emphasis	Individuality
Extended family	Nuclear/blended family
Person-to-person orientation	Person-to-object orientation
Acceptance/resignation	Aggression/assertion
Fatalism	Self-determination
Present orientation	Future orientation

expected to expand to 40.2 million (13.4% of the population) by 2010 (American Demographics, 1991).

Although the largest group of blacks is of African descent, some blacks trace their recent ancestry—and consequently their cultural identity—to nations in the Caribbean. In some areas, blacks refer to themselves as Eritreans, Kenyans, African Americans, Haitians, or Dominicans (from the Dominican Republic).

Terms for black Americans have evolved over the twentieth century from *colored* to *Negro* to *black*, to *Afro-American*, to **African American**, a term that became popular after it was used in 1988 by Jesse Jackson. Many black Americans prefer the term *African American* to *black* because of its emphasis on heritage rather than color (Barnhart & Metcalf, 1999). However, the name *African American* does not encompass the thousands of black Americans whose recent ancestry is from areas other than Africa, such as the Caribbean.

Some black Americans do have different values from what we refer to as mainstream white American values. Unlike mainstream white Americans, however, many blacks experienced and struggled against racism perpetuated by both white individuals and institutions. In some ways, many blacks have adopted values that reflect their experiences in an environment dominated by white culture. Because of a perceived need for solidarity, some blacks seek the solace and strength that lie in the family, church, and black community.

Blacks traditionally have been more present oriented than whites. Some blacks still focus on the present because they believe the future will contain the same elements of racism and discrimination that oppressed them in the past. Other blacks actively plan for the future and strive for higher education and professional status.

Although many of us have a stereotypic view of a dominant female figure as the head of black households, a woman's role varies depending on the family. In some families, the mother, grandmother, or aunt is the primary caregiver for several children; however, families vary in their composition and in the roles assumed by family members.

Table 2-3 summarizes some common differences in the traditional values of black and white American cultures. As you review Table 2-3, remember that individuals may or may not choose to follow the traditional values of their culture. Also, people who belong to different cultures but share similar educational, economic, and occupational backgrounds will likely share similar values. For example, blacks and whites who graduate from a university and pursue professional careers may also share similar values concerning financial security, family, childrearing, and education.

◆◆◆◆ **TABLE 2-3** ◆◆◆◆

**Examples of Values of Blacks Primarily from
Black Communities and
Values of Mainstream White Americans**

Values Common to Blacks	Values Common to Mainstream Whites
Family bonding	Individualism
Matrifocus	Patrifocus
Present oriented	Future oriented
Spiritual orientation	Personal mastery

Native American Values

Native Americans (American Indians) are a highly heterogeneous group, constituting 0.9% of the total U.S. population (U.S. Census Bureau, 2001c), including approximately 530 tribal groups. According to the 1990 U.S. Census and the *Source Book of Zip Code Demographics*, the five largest Native American communities or cultural nations in the lower forty-eight states were:

1. Cherokee, 369,035 people.

2. Navajo, 225,298 people.

3. Chippewa, 105,988 people.

4. Sioux, 107,321 people.

5. Choctaw, 82,231 people.

The 1990 U.S. Census also reported that the Native American population of Alaska is composed of:

- 21,869 American Indian/Athapaskan people who live in both Alaska and Canada.

- 10,052 Aleuts who inhabit the Aleutian Islands and the Alaskan peninsula.

- 44,400 Eskimos who primarily live near the Bering Sea and Arctic Ocean coasts (Lefever & Davidhizar, 1995).

Most Native Americans are burdened with poverty. For example, on the Navajo reservation, only 60% of homes have adequate plumbing or a bedroom or are hooked to a public sewer system; only 23% of homes have a telephone; only 6% use electricity for heat. Typically, wood serves as the major heating fuel for a reservation home (1990 Census of Population Characteristics of American Indians by Tribe and Language, 1994).

According to the U.S. Department of Housing and Urban Development–U.S. Census Bureau, 30% of Native Americans live below the poverty line, compared with 29.5% of blacks, 25.3% of Hispanics, 14.1% of Asian/Pacific Islanders, and 9.8% of whites. Also, Native Americans have the lowest life expectancy of any ethnic group in the United States. Native Americans can expect to live only two-thirds as long as other people in the United States.

Many Native American families take pride in maintaining a traditional lifestyle and prefer the ways of their grandparents. They may not want to embrace all the values of mainstream American culture. There are many variations in family patterns of blending mainstream values and urban ways, with traditional values and what some term *Indian ways*.

Traditional culture can give individual Native Americans security and a sense of belonging. Members who decide to leave the reservation to pursue opportunities in the broader world outside may suffer from a loss of identity, as traditional values clash with new lifestyles.

Example: When a white, middle-class youth decides to go away to college, proud parents may view this action as a welcome sign that their child is ambitious and goal oriented. When a Native American youth leaves the reservation to seek a college education, elders may interpret this action in many ways: they may see the youth as relinquishing identity with family and community members, as acquiring different values, or as preparing to help or care for other Native Americans.

Many Native Americans value the extended family. Thus, grandparents, aunts, and uncles—even though they live in separate households—are actively involved in raising the children. Women play a major role in working with and educating youth.

Other Native American values include:

- The importance of sharing one's worldly goods with others rather than hoarding possessions.
- Cooperating with others, rather than competing against others.
- Working for the good of the group, rather than for the good of the individual.
- Respecting the rights of others, rather than interfering with others.
- Being involved with the present rather than with the future.
- Accepting nature and the natural order of things, rather than trying to control nature.

Table 2-4 summarizes some differences in the traditional values of Native Americans and mainstream white Americans.

◆◆◆◆ **TABLE 2-4** ◆◆◆◆

Examples of Values of Native Americans Who Primarily Live on Reservations and Values of Mainstream White Americans

Values Common to Some Native Americans	Values Common To Some Mainstream Whites
Bonding to family or group	Individualism
Sharing with others	Accumulating for self
Present orientation	Future orientation
Extended family	Nuclear family
Cooperation	Competition
Acceptance of nature	Mastery over nature

VALUES OF OTHER SELECTED AMERICAN CULTURAL GROUPS

Although the five broad cultural groups just discussed have had an enormous impact on American values, there are many other important cultural groups that have immigrated to the New World, bringing their values with them. Indeed, the United States is a land that has been built, in large part, by immigrants. Since the early 1700s, hundreds of thousands of immigrants fleeing from poverty, war, and religious persecution have come to this nation in search of wealth and freedom. Immigrants have come from all over the world—Europe, the British Isles, the Middle East, Asia, India, and the Philippines—to help build the American way of life. Because of space limitations, this section discusses the values of only five of the many vital cultures that have settled in the United States: the Amish, Filipinos, Iranians, Irish, and Jews.

Amish Values

The **Old Order Amish** (pronounced ah-mish) is an ethnoreligious group that migrated from Germany to the United States almost 300 years ago. As did other groups of immigrants, the Amish came to the New World in search of religious freedom. Between 1900 and 1996, the Old Order Amish population grew from 5000 to over 100,000 people (Brewer & Bonalumi, 1996).

COMMUNICATION CONSIDERATIONS

The Amish are distinguished by their strict adherence to their traditional values and their resistance to acculturation into the white mainstream culture that surrounds them.

The Amish, who choose to live in rural farming areas, have developed settlements in more than twenty states. However, approximately 75% of their total population reside in Pennsylvania, Ohio, and Indiana. Amish settlements are divided into church districts that are composed of thirty to forty families. Because church districts are only about 3 miles apart, it is easy for Amish families to travel between districts by horse and buggy, their traditional mode of transportation.

Love of family is at the center of the Amish person's life. Ideally, the three-generational Amish family is composed of the father, mother, seven children, and the grandparents, who help provide child care. Although the man is the head of the family, women are respected in their roles of wife and mother. Although marriages between first cousins are discouraged, the Amish tend to marry among themselves, a practice that has lead to genetic disorders (Wenger, 1991).

As a group, the Amish strive in every way to insulate themselves and their children from worldly influences. Access to print and electronic media is restricted. Although the Amish may publish their own newsletters, they avoid exposure to secular newspapers, radio and television programs, and the Internet. Children are educated only through the eighth grade, and then they are expected to engage in productive work on the farm. Although English is used in Amish schools, the Amish prefer to use **Deitsch**, or Pennsylvania German, when at home and in the community.

The Amish also dress in a manner that clearly sets them apart from other people. Homemade clothing is characterized by its plain old-fashioned designs and somber colors. Women do not wear jewelry or cosmetics; they wear their long hair braided or pinned under a white organdy cap, which is topped with a black bonnet for outdoor wear.

Important Amish traditional values include the following (Wenger & Wenger, 2003):

- **Demut**, which is German for "humility." This value is expressed in the plain dress and modest demeanor of the Amish in public.
- **Gelassenheit**. This term is German for "passiveness," "quiet acceptance of life," and "contentment."

- *Caring for the needs of others.* This value, especially caring for those who are ill or elderly, is paramount. Helping others is the *Amish Way*.

- *Conformity to the will of the group.* This value is far more important than individual rights. The Amish are cooperative, not competitive, with each other.

Filipino Values

Filipinos are the fastest growing Asian group in North America, with a U.S. population of 1,450,000 and a Canadian population of 157,250 people (Pacquiao, 2003). Most of the Filipinos in the United States have immigrated from the Philippine Islands, which are located in the Pacific Ocean, approximately 450 miles from the coast of China.

Over the centuries, the culture of the Philippines has been influenced by the Malaysian, Chinese, Japanese, Indonesian, and Asian Indian cultures. Philippine culture was also shaped by the Arabs, who brought Islam to the Islands in the late 1300s, and later by the Spaniards, who converted the majority of Filipinos to Catholicism. In addition, American servicemen who were stationed in the Philippines during World War II brought American ideas and values to the Filipino people (Pacquiao, 2003).

Tagalog is the primary language spoken in the Philippines. The two other official languages are English and Spanish. However, within the Philippines there are approximately seventy-five ethnolinguistic groups, who speak more than 100 languages. For the sake of simplicity, the Philippine government has given all of these languages the collective name of **Pilipino**.

The Filipino family is basically monogamous, although some **Muslim** Filipinos believe in polygamy. Husbands are titular heads of the household, but mothers have an equal say in decisions regarding family finances and the children. Because education paves the road to better jobs and higher salaries, Filipino families vigorously promote higher education for their children. Fathers and mothers willingly sacrifice to send their older children to school. The older children are then expected to help younger siblings obtain a sound education. Filipino Americans also want their children to learn Western ways in order to successfully blend in with the dominant white culture in America.

Traditional Filipino values include the following (Pacquiao, 2003):

- **Galang** or respect, is the primary Filipino value. In particular, Filipinos must honor and respect their parents and elders. For example, it is important to avoid openly disagreeing with a parent or older sibling. A Filipino nurse who emigrates to the United States may find it difficult to disagree with an administrator or physician (see Chapter 14). A person who is not respectful loses face and suffers *hiya*, or shame.

- **Amor propio** is having personal pride, saving face, and avoiding hiya. One way by which Filipinos save face is to avoid arguing with older people and individuals in authority.

- *Acceptance of pain and suffering* is considered honorable. Some Filipinos believe that pain provides an opportunity for spiritual growth.

Iranian Values

Approximately 1 million Iranians currently live in the United States. Around 450,000 Iranians live in California; 39,000 reside in Canada. Los Angeles contains the largest population of Iranians in the world outside of Iran (Hafizi & Lipson, 2003).

From 1980 to 1992, an estimated 800,000 Iranians emigrated to the United States from Iran, formerly known as Persia. Most of these Iranian immigrants were fleeing the aftermath of the 1979 Islamic revolution and the 1980s war between Iran and Iraq (Pliskin, 1992).

Unfortunately, because of anti-American events in Iran, Iranian refugees have been subjected to ethnic bias and discrimination in the United States. Anti-Iranian sentiments ran particularly high in this country as a result of the Hostage Crisis, during which a U.S. embassy in Tehran was occupied between November 1979 and January 1981 by followers of the Ayatollah Khomeini. Being forced to flee from a revolution at home to a new country where they were disliked and distrusted adversely affected many Iranians, both physically and emotionally.

Despite these problems, Iranian immigrants (many from upper and middle class backgrounds) have been able to create a middle-class lifestyle for themselves in the United States. In the ethnic community in Los Angeles, many Iranians who were formerly physicians, engineers, or professors in Iran have gone into business for themselves. In 1987, 61% of Iranians in Los Angeles were self-employed. Many opened their own pizza parlor or gas station or owned their own taxicab. Iranian women developed home-based businesses, working as seamstresses, pastry makers, beauticians, or makeup artists. Iranians have tended to avoid menial labor, because this type of work is not respected in Iran (Hafizi & Lipson, 2003).

Although the majority of Iranians who have come to the United States are Muslims, small groups of Iranians embrace Judaism, Christianity,

Baha'is, and Zorasterism. Strict Muslims observe Friday as a holy day, and they strive to practice the five tenets of the Islamic faith:

1. Believe in Allah.
2. Pray five times a day at designated times.
3. Give to the poor.
4. Fast during the month of Ramadan.
5. Make a once-in-a-lifetime pilgrimage to the holy city of Mecca in Saudi Arabia.

Many Iranian Americans do not observe all of the traditional practices of Islam.

The Iranian family is patriarchal and hierarchical. The father is the head of the household, and he expects his wife and children to obey him. In the father's absence, the oldest son is in control. Although the status of Iranian women has improved since the 1960s' social reforms in Iran, wives are still expected to defer to their husbands and care for the home and children, even though they may be working outside the home.

Traditional Iranian values include the following:

- *Respect for higher education and advanced degrees.* Iranians are among the most highly educated immigrants in the United States.

- **Zerangi**, or *cleverness*. Iranians respect the person who is able to barter and bargain in the marketplace and, consequently, get the highest price possible.

- *Respect for elders.* Iranians feel that they are obligated to take care of their elderly relatives.

- *Respect for Persia's religious and artistic heritage.* Persia has produced some of the world's greatest art and poetry. Persia has also contributed to the disciplines of philosophy and medicine.

- *Modesty, respectability, and politeness.* Iranians believe that it is important to please others, be hospitable, and maintain a good reputation.

Irish Values

Irish traditions and values are a major part of American culture. Millions of Irish have emigrated to the United States over the last four centuries. Today, it is estimated that one in every five people in the United States is of Irish descent. In other words, 38.7 million people or 15.6% of the population can proudly claim an Irish heritage (Wilson, 2003).

The majority of Irish Americans emigrated to the United States from Ireland (Eire) between the 1600s and 1965. The Irish left their homeland to escape religious persecution, extreme poverty, and the constant threat of famine. The first settlers made their home in the northeastern part of this country. For this reason, Boston, Philadelphia, and New York contain the largest Irish settlements in the United States. During the 1920s, 90% of the Irish lived in the cities, and they became known as the **Shanty Irish**. Later, many of the second- and third-generational Irish moved to the suburbs, where they became known as the **Lace Curtain Irish**.

Although the Irish suffered greatly in their homeland, life in the New World was also difficult for the new immigrants. The early Irish settlers were persecuted for their Roman Catholic faith. The majority lived hard lives in poverty. However, a strong religious faith, work ethic, and sense of humor helped the Irish survive the harsh early years in this country and successfully assimilate into the mainstream white culture.

The traditional Irish family is patrilineal, although modern Irish families are more democratic, with all members willing to share household and childrearing tasks. Because of their strong sense of tradition, the Irish tend to be oriented toward the past. Also, the Irish are traditionally fatalistic. Many Irish believe that humans are subject to the laws of nature and of God, and thus there is little a person can do to correct a problem. This belief may explain why some Irish tend to deny and ignore illnesses and pain.

Traditional Irish values include the following:

- *Obligation and devotion to the family.* Traditionally, the Irish have valued large families with many children.

- *Strong faith in God.* The majority of Irish Americans are Roman Catholics.

- *Respect for the elderly.* The Irish value the advice and experience of the elderly.

- *Education and hard work.* The Irish are well represented in law, medicine, science, and literature. The Irish have also risen to prominence in politics.

- *Accepting life's difficulties with humor.* The Irish are known for their humor, wit, and ability to write biting social satire.

Jewish Values

The word *Jew* is defined in *Webster's Dictionary* as "(1) one who is descended or regarded as descended from the ancient Hebrews, and (2) one whose religion is Judaism." The practice of Judaism ranges from liberal Reform to

Orthodox. Orthodox Jews recognize the child who is born to a Jewish mother as a Jew. **Reform Jews** are more liberal, and they also recognize the child who is born to a Jewish father and a non-Jewish mother as Jewish (Selekman, 2003).

Jewish people do not belong to a race, nor do they belong to any one nationality. People who call themselves Jews come from all over the world. **Ashkenazi** (Yiddish for "German") **Jews** come from Eastern Europe and Russia; 82% of Jews are of Ashkenazi descent. **Sephardic Jews** come from Spain, Portugal, the Mediterranean area, Africa, Central America, and South America. **Sabras** are Jews born in Israel.

Although the Jewish people have highly diverse backgrounds, Jews also have a great deal in common. Jews share religious beliefs, cultural values, family traditions, and common folk traditions. Jews also share a long and painful history of persecution. The Jewish people have suffered tremendous losses of life, liberty, and property during, for example, the anti-Jewish riots (**pogroms**) in Russia and Eastern Europe, and the **Holocaust** in Nazi Germany and Poland. Even those Jews who emigrated to the United States in search of freedom and peace faced prejudice and anti-Semitism in their new homeland.

Approximately 5.7 million Jews (around 1% of the world Jewish population) live in the United States (Selekman, 2003). The Jewish immigrants primarily settled in the Northeast. Today, Jews live in large cities all over this country: for example, Los Angeles, New York, Miami, and Boston. As a group, Jewish Americans have attained professional respect and economic success. Because the Jews greatly value higher education and advanced degrees, many Jewish Americans are professional people who excel as lawyers, physicians, dentists, scientists, and university professors.

In addition to education and work, Jewish life revolves around religion and family life. Judaism is a **monotheistic** faith (belief in one God) primarily based on the **Torah**, or first five books of the Bible, also known as the Books of Moses. The rabbi is the spiritual leader of the Jews. Jewish services are held in a synagogue, temple, or shul, where prayer is conducted in Hebrew. In the United States, Judaism is divided into three major denominations:

1. **Orthodox Jews** adhere strictly to the traditions of Judaism, the traditional Code of Jewish Law, and dietary laws that state which foods are **kosher** (fit for eating) and which foods are **treyf** (forbidden or unclean). **Hasidic Jews** are ultra-Orthodox traditionalists who rigidly follow strict rules in their dress, living arrangements, and religious practices.

2. **Conservative Jews** follow many of the Orthodox Jewish traditions but are less strict in their adherence to Jewish mores.

3. *Reform Jews* are much more liberal in their beliefs and practices than Orthodox and Conservative Jews. For example, Reform Jews may not observe traditional dietary practices.

Jewish family life depends upon which branch of Judaism is practiced by family members. Traditional or Orthodox Jewish families are definitely male-oriented, whereas the families of Conservative and Reform Jews are more equalitarian. Jewish marriages are monogamous. Jewish parents welcome children as blessings, and they strive to provide their offspring with love, a religious upbringing, and an excellent education.

Traditional Jewish values include the following:

- *Higher education and continued learning throughout life.*

- **Tzedakah**, or righteousness and sharing. Jewish people value being charitable and generous toward persons in need.

- *Respect for parents and elders.* Jews believe that it is important to honor their fathers and mothers and to care for their elderly parents and relatives.

- *Modesty and humility.* These virtues are particularly valued by Orthodox Jews.

- *Humor.* Jews value the ability to laugh at a situation and at themselves as a way to cope with bias and prejudice.

- *Good health.* When ill, Jews value regaining their health to such a degree that they may waive traditional practices (such as dietary laws) if these practices might interfere with the healing process.

REFERENCES

American Demographics Inc. (1991). American diversity: What the 1990 Census reveals about population growth, blacks, Hispanics, Asians, ethnic diversity, and children—and what it means to you. *American Demographics Desk Reference Series*, No 1.

Andrews, M. M., & Boyle, J. S. (2002). *Transcultural concepts in nursing care* (4th ed.). Philadelphia: Lippincott.

Barnhart, D. K., & Metcalf, A. (1999). *America in so many words: Words that have shaped America*. Boston: Houghton Mifflin.

Brewer, J. A., & Bonalumi, N. M. (1996). Cultural diversity in the emergency department: Health care beliefs and practices among the Pennsylvania Amish. *Journal of Emergency Nursing, 21*(6), 494–497.

Compton's Interactive Encyclopedia. Copyright © 1994, 1995, 1996, Compton's NewMedia, Inc.

Hafizi, H., & Lipson, J. G. (2003). Iranian heritage. In L. D. Purnell & B. J. Paulanka (Eds.), *Transcultural health care: A culturally competent approach* (2nd ed.). Philadelphia: Davis.

Holmes, S. A. (1998). Blacks consider new face of race issues. *Seattle Times*, p. 47.

Lefever, D., & Davidhizar, R. E. (1995). American Eskimos. In J. N. Giger & R. E. Davidhizer (Eds.), *Transcultural nursing: Assessment and intervention* (2nd ed.). St. Louis: Mosby.

Miller, S. W., & Goodin, J. N. (1995). East Indian Hindu Americans. In J. N. Giger & R. E. Davidhizar (Eds.), *Transcultural nursing: Assessment and intervention* (2nd ed.). St. Louis: Mosby.

Pacquiao, D. F. (2003). Filipino heritage. In L. D. Purnell & B. J. Paulanka (Eds.), *Transcultural health care: A culturally competent approach* (2nd ed.). Philadelphia: Davis.

Pliskin, K. L. (1992). Dysphoria and somatization in Iranian culture (Cross-cultural medicine—A decade later). [Special issue]. *The Western Journal of Medicine, 157*, 295–300.

Selekman, J. (2003). Jewish heritage. In L. D. Purnell & B. J. Paulanka (Eds.), *Transcultural health care: A culturally competent approach* (2nd ed). Philadelphia: Davis.

Spector, R. E. (2004). *Cultural diversity in health and illness* (6th ed.). Upper Saddle River, NJ: Pearson Prentice Hall.

Sue, D. W., & Sue, D. (1990). *Counseling the culturally different: Theory and practice* (2nd ed.). New York: Wiley.

U.S. Census Bureau. (2001a). The Asian population: 2000. U.S. Department of Commerce. Retrieved March 7, 2002. From: *www.census.gov*. Press Release 2001.

U.S. Census Bureau. (2001b). Census 2000 paints statistical portrait of the nation's Hispanic population. U.S. Department of Commerce. Retrieved March 7, 2002. From: *www.census.gov*. Press Release 2001.

U.S. Census Bureau. (2001c). Census 2000 shows America's diversity. U.S. Department of Commerce. Retrieved March 7, 2002. From: *www.census.gov*. Press Release 2001.

Watts, A. (1999). *The way of Zen.* Part of the vintage spiritual classics series. Vintage Publishers.

Wenger, A. F. Z. (1991). Culture-specific care and the Old Order Amish. *NSNA Imprint, 38*(2), 80–93.

Wenger, A. F. Z., & Wenger, M. R. (2003). The Amish. In L. D. Purnell & B. J. Paulanka (Eds.), *Transcultural health care: A culturally competent approach* (2nd ed.). Philadelphia: Davis.

Wilson, S. A. (2003). Irish heritage. In L. D. Purnell & B. J. Paulanka (Eds.), *Transcultural health care: A culturally competent approach* (2nd ed.). Philadelphia: Davis.

Zehavi, A. M. (Ed.). (1973). *Handbook of the world's religions.* New York: Franklin Watts.

Zich, A. (1991, November). Japan's sun rises over the Pacific. *National Geographic,* pp. 35–66.

SUGGESTED READINGS

Axtell, R. E. (Ed.). (1993). *Do's and taboos around the world* (3rd ed.). New York: Wiley.

Edmission, K. W. (1997). Psychosocial dimensions of medical-surgical nursing. In J. M. Black & E. Matassarin-Jacobs (Eds.), *Medical surgical nursing: Clinical management for continuity of care.* Philadelphia: Saunders.

Intuit. *Microsoft® Encarta® Encyclopedia* © 1993–1996. Microsoft Corporation. All rights reserved.

Lee, E. (Ed.). (2000). *Working with Asian Americans: A guide for clinicians.* New York: Guilford Press.

Lipson, J. G. (1992). The health and adjustment of Iranian immigrants. *Western Journal of Nursing Research, 14*(1),10–29.

Martin, C. (2003). Irish Americans. In J. N. Giger & R. E. Davidhizar (Eds.), *Transcultural nursing: Assessment and intervention* (4th ed.). St. Louis: Mosby.

Meleis, A. I. (1997). Immigrant transitions and health care: An action plan [News]. *Nursing Outlook, 45*(1), 42.

Native Americans. *Microsoft® Encarta® Encyclopedia* © 1993–1996. Microsoft Corporation. All rights reserved.

Porter, C. P., & Villarruel, A. M. (1993). Nursing research with African American and Hispanic people: Guidelines for action. *Nursing Outlook, 41*(2), 59–67.

Schwartz, E. A. (2003). Jewish Americans. In J. N. Giger & R. E. Davidhizar (Eds.), *Transcultural nursing: Assessment and intervention* (4th ed.). St. Louis: Mosby.

Smitherman, G. (1994). *Black talk: Words and phrases from the hood to the amen corner.* Boston: Houghton Mifflin.

Sutherland, D., & Morris, B. J. (1996). Caring for the Islamic patient. *Journal of Emergency Nursing, 21*(6), 508–509.

Vance, A. R. (2003). Filipino heritage. In J. N. Giger & R. E. Davidhizar (Eds.), *Transcultural nursing: Assessment and intervention* (4th ed.). St. Louis: Mosby.

CHAPTER 3

Enhancing Transcultural Communication through Culturally Competent and Linguistically Appropriate Services

KEY TERMS

- CLAS Standards
- Cultural Awareness
- Cultural Competence
- Cultural Desire
- Cultural Encounter
- Cultural Knowledge
- Cultural & Linguistic Competence
- Cultural Skill

OBJECTIVES

After completing this chapter, you should be able to:

- Define cultural competence.
- Describe the various components of the Process of Cultural Competence.
- Identify the Standards for Culturally and Linguistically Appropriate Services.
- Discuss the relevance of the CLAS standards to professional practice.

INTRODUCTION

Developing cultural competency is a professional expectation for all health care practitioners. Because culture and communication are strongly linked and the population needing health care services has become increasingly diverse, nurses need to demonstrate core knowledge and skills in providing care for clients with different cultural backgrounds and with limited English proficiency. It is important that all health care providers respond with respect and sensitivity when interacting with clients and families from different cultural and linguistic backgrounds. Leininger and McFarland (2002) stressed the importance of cultural care competency for diverse cultures and commonalities. Furthermore, they stated that nurses need to be knowledgeable about their own cultural heritage and of their biases, beliefs, and practices to provide sensitive and effective nursing care. Barriers to health care can be linguistic and cultural. For example, a client who does not believe in biomedical or scientific explanations of illness and disease will find it difficult to comply with the treatment regimen. If the client does not speak English, interpreters' services need to be provided so that effective communication is achieved. Errors in communication can lead to misdiagnosis or inappropriate treatment. Positive outcomes of cultural competency in practice have been clearly demonstrated in improving the quality of health care services, increasing client satisfaction, decreasing errors in practice, increasing clients' compliance to prescribed treatment regimens, and reducing liability and malpractice suits. Clearly, clients who do not understand the treatment they are receiving are not likely to comply with it.

As the United States continues to become increasingly multiethnic and culturally diverse, standards of cultural competency in the service professions are desirable. In fact, cultural competence is synonymous with nursing competence because nurses need to plan care on the basis of individualized and personalized needs. The goal of cultural competence is to "minimize cultural dissonance and improve patient–provider communication, thus reducing opportunities for errors, increasing compliance and producing better clinical outcomes" (Dreher & MacNaughton, 2002). Furthermore, they pointed out that nurses need to carefully examine intragroup and intergroup variations or differences to avoid the pitfall of stereotyping client responses. Nurses need to utilize cultural knowledge in planning care but must assess the client to ensure that the cultural information is true and is validated during the nurse–client encounter.

THE IMPORTANCE OF CULTURAL COMPETENCE IN THE NURSE–PATIENT RELATIONSHIP

The concept of cultural competence has been explored quite extensively in current literature and has been emphasized as a professional imperative for nurses in providing care to an ethnic and racially diverse client population. Transcultural communication is clearly a core component of cultural competency. The American Nurses Association (ANA) position statement (1991) and the American Academy of Nursing (1992) have recognized cultural competency as a professional responsibility in providing care. The ANA position paper on cultural diversity in nursing practice stressed the importance of considering specific cultural factors and cultural differences in assessing the needs of clients and families of diverse backgrounds. Furthermore, it pointed out that nurses in clinical practice must use their knowledge of cross-cultural communication to develop and implement culturally sensitive and linguistically appropriate nursing care. Recognizing differences, integrating cultural knowledge, and acting in a culturally appropriate manner will facilitate cultural competence. Campinha-Bacote (1999) defined cultural competence as a process in which the nurse who is involved with the client and the family continuously strives to provide culturally competent care. There are five components in the Process of Cultural Competence Model (Campinha-Bacote & Muñoz, 2001) in the delivery of health care services: (1) cultural awareness, (2) cultural knowledge, (3) cultural skill, (4) cultural encounter, and (5) cultural desire. Campinha-Bacote defines these components as follows.

Cultural awareness is the deliberate cognitive process in which the nurse appreciates and is sensitive to the cultural values of the client. This also includes an awareness of the health care provider's cultural beliefs, values, and practices. The goal is for a heightened awareness of one's cultural background that may influence the cross-cultural communication process. Effective communication may not be reached if the nurse is not aware of his or her own biases and prejudices against individuals of different ethnic and cultural backgrounds. The following questions may enhance the level of self-awareness:

1. What is your cultural heritage?
2. Do you identify with a specific ethnic group?
3. What are some of your experiences with people who are different?
4. What personal characteristics do you have that will help you establish a professional helping relationship with ethnically diverse clients and families?

5. What personal characteristics do you have that will be detrimental to establishing a professional helping relationship with ethnically diverse clients and families?

Cultural knowledge consists of the sound educational foundation in which the nurse gathers cultural information in a formal or informal manner that may include world views of different cultures, values, and beliefs as well as perceptions about health and illness. World view, the individual's perception of the world, is greatly influenced by one's cultural background and life experiences. Therefore, it is important for the nurse to understand and assess the client's health belief system and world view. For example, an individual may believe that illness is due to a magic spell or hex that someone with magical powers has cast upon the individual. This magico-religious paradigm is widely accepted in some traditional Hispanic, Caribbean, Asian, and African cultures. Cultural knowledge also includes an understanding of the biological variations that are found in clients with different cultural background. For example, nurses need to recognize the fact that there are specific ethnic and cultural differences in drug response as well as variations in the clinical significance of certain laboratory tests such as glucose levels, values of hemoglobin, and hematocrit.

Cultural skill is the ability to collect relevant cultural data through interviews to obtain the client's health history and presenting problem. Various culturological assessment tools have been developed to gather data about the ethnic and cultural values and beliefs of the client. Communication styles and meanings become very important in gathering cultural data in the assessment process. Expressions of verbal and nonverbal messages are culturally influenced. The majority group tends to be open, disclosing, and willing to share their thoughts and feelings with others. In some cultural groups, clients may not be readily willing to self-disclose. For example, most Native Americans are very private and, therefore, may not volunteer a lot of personal information as readily as other groups.

The nurse also needs to consider communication patterns when planning care, such as high-context and low-context communication patterns. The high-context groups emphasize the importance of nonverbal expressions, gestures, posture, and eye contact in relation to the environment and in giving an accurate meaning to the message expressed verbally. The high-context group includes Asians, African Americans, and Native Americans. The focus of communication in the low-context group is verbal articulation and verbal expressions. The expectation is that the individual clearly shares feelings and thoughts through precise verbal expressions. The environment and nonverbal messages are secondary to the words expressed.

Communication is so complex in the patient–provider relationship that it is extremely important to recognize the potential problem with a non-English-speaking client. Because there may be several languages or dialects that clients and their families speak, it is best for the health care provider to obtain a formally trained, preferably certified, interpreter.

Cultural encounter is the process in which the nurse seeks opportunities to engage in cross-cultural interactions directly or indirectly. A direct cultural encounter occurs when the nurse provides direct care to a client from a different cultural background, utilizing cultural knowledge and implementing cultural skill in the care provided. An indirect encounter occurs when the nurse obtains cultural information based on the experiences of another nurse in a direct encounter. For example, the nurse who is taking care of a client from Somalia may be able to share with other health care providers some of the health beliefs and practices held by this group as well as insight into the refugee experience. Nurses and other health care providers are encouraged to seek opportunities to have cultural encounters and cultural interactions with individuals with diverse ethnic and cultural backgrounds.

Cultural desire is the genuine and sincere desire to work effectively with minority clients and their families. This motivation to want to provide care that is sensitive and appropriate is reflective of the caring that health care providers demonstrate in providing services. Cultural desire can be achieved only if the individual wants to engage in the process of cultural competence.

NATIONAL STANDARDS FOR CLAS IN HEALTH CARE

The national standards for Culturally and Linguistically Appropriate Services (CLAS) were developed by the U.S. Department of Health and Human Services, Office of Minority Health, and appeared in the *Federal Register* in December 2000. The standards were intended to include all cultures and are not limited to a specific population or ethnic group. The process of developing these standards started with an analytical review of numerous regulations, contracts, key legislation, and standards that were currently being used by various health care agencies across the country. This effort basically was in response to the increasing need to ensure that the recipients of health care services are provided equitable and effective treatment. These standards were proposed to address the inequities that currently exist in the provision of health care services to people of color. Ethnic and racial health disparities have been well documented and have existed in the health care delivery system for a long time. Clearly, health disparities continue to affect a disproportionate number of people of color. The CLAS standards hope to address this well-known issue of health disparities. It also addresses the various definitions and interpretations of the meaning and implementation of cultural competency by developing one universally understood set of standards. The goal is to ultimately improve the health status of all Americans and to contribute to the elimination of racial and ethnic health disparities that most minorities experience in the health care system in this country.

The following definition of **cultural competence**, adapted from Cross, Bazron, and co-workers (1989) was the overarching definition that guided the development of the CLAS standards:

> **Cultural and linguistic competence** is a set of congruent behaviors, attitudes, and policies that come together in a system, agency, or among professionals that enables effective work in cross-cultural situations.

> *Culture* refers to integrated patterns of human behavior that includes the language, thoughts, communication, actions, customs, beliefs, values, and institutions of racial, ethnic, religious, or social groups.

> *Competence* implies having the capacity to function effectively as an individual and an organization within the context of the cultural beliefs, behaviors, and needs presented by consumers and their communities.

CLAS standards are primarily directed at health care organizations. Unfortunately, there is a lack of consensus and guidance as to what cultural competency means for a particular organization. Health care organizations are strongly encouraged to use the standards as a framework in providing culturally and linguistically appropriate services and to integrate CLAS activities throughout their organization in collaboration with the communities they serve. For example, a Hispanic interpreter needs to be available to provide language assistance services if the organization serves a Hispanic community.

Other than nurses and other health care providers, the following groups may use CLAS standards to guide them:

> *Clients and families* need to be able to understand their right to receive respectful and appropriate health care services in their primary language.

> *Professional organizations* may use them to guide their standards of practice. Examples include the American Nurses Association, the

American Medical Association, the American Academy of Pediatrics, the National Association of Social Work, and the Liaison Committee on Medical Education.

Accrediting agencies use them to guide the accreditation standards. Examples include the Joint Commission of Healthcare Organizations (JCAHO) and the National Committee on Quality Assurance (NCQA) and other peer review and quality review organizations.

Policy makers, including all federal, state, and local legislators, can use them to draft laws and regulations for providing culturally competent health care services.

Educators in the human service professions—such as nursing, medicine, social work, education, and other legal and social service professions—can use them to incorporate curricular content on cultural competence.

Client advocates use them to promote access to quality health care for diverse populations.

Members of the community being served use them to assess the relevance and applicability of the standards in their specific communities.

The fourteen **CLAS standards** are organized by themes (Table 3-1): *Culturally Competent Care (Standards 1–3)* refers to the professional relationship between the health care provider, who provides culturally competent care, and the client or recipient of these services. *Language Access Services (Standards 4–7)* focuses on the role of the health care provider in ensuring that language access services are provided. *Organizational Supports for Cultural Competence (Standards 8–14)* focuses on the role of health care providers within the system in supporting and maintaining standards in their organizations.

These standards may be mandates, recommendations, or guidelines. For example, all recipients of federal funds are mandated to meet standards 4, 5, 6, and 7, requiring language assistance services to all clients with Limited English Proficiency (LEP). Title VI of the Civil Rights Act of 1964 states that "no person in the United States shall, on the grounds of race, color or national origin be excluded from participation in, denied the benefits of, or be otherwise subjected to discrimination" while receiving services from a federally supported program" (Office of Civil Rights, 2000).

The U.S. Department of Health and Human Services' (DHHS) Office of Civil Rights views the lack of interpreter services for individuals with limited English proficiency as a form of discrimination; therefore, all DHHS-funded programs are required to provide interpreters at no cost to the client.

◆◆◆◆ ▓▓▓▓▓▓ **TABLE 3-1** ▓▓▓▓▓▓ ◆◆◆◆

Standards for Culturally and Linguistically Appropriate Services (CLAS)

Standard 1. Health care organizations should ensure that the patients/consumers receive from all staff members effective, understandable, and respectful care that is provided in a manner compatible with their cultural health beliefs and practices and preferred language.

Standard 2. Health care organizations should implement strategies to recruit, retain, and promote at all levels of the organization a diverse staff and leadership that are representative of the demographic characteristics of the service area.

Standard 3. Health care organizations should ensure that staff at all levels and across all disciplines receive ongoing education and training in culturally and linguistically appropriate service delivery.

Standard 4. Health care organizations must offer and provide language assistance services, at no cost, to each patient/consumer with limited English proficiency at all points of contact in a timely manner during all hours of operation.

Standard 5. Health care organizations must provide to patients/consumers in their preferred language both verbal offers and written notices informing them of their right to receive language assistance services.

Standard 6. Health care organizations must ensure the competence of language assistance provided to limited English proficient patients/consumers by interpreters and bilingual staff. Family and friends should not be used to provide interpretation services (except on request by the patient/consumer).

Standard 7. Health care organizations must make available easily understood patient-related materials and post signage in the language of the commonly encountered group or groups represented in the service area.

Standard 8. Health care organizations should develop, implement, and promote a written strategic plan that outlines clear goals, policies and operational plans, and management accountability/oversight mechanisms to provide culturally and linguistically appropriate services.

Standard 9. Health care organizations should conduct initial and ongoing organizational self-assessments of CLAS-related activities and are encouraged to integrate cultural and linguistic competence-related measures into their internal audits, performance improvement programs, patient satisfaction assessments, and outcome-based evaluations.

Standard 10. Health care organizations should ensure that data on the individual patient's/consumer's race, ethnicity, and spoken and written language are collected in health records, integrated into the organization's management information systems, and periodically updated.

Standard 11. Health care organizations should maintain a current demographic, cultural, and epidemiological profile of the community as well as a needs assessment to accurately plan for and implement services that respond to the cultural and linguistic characteristics of the service area.

Standard 12. Health care should develop participatory, collaborative partnerships with communities and utilize a variety of formal and informal mechanisms to facilitate community and patient/consumer involvement in designing and implementing CLAS-related activities.

Standard 13. Health care organizations should ensure that conflict and grievance resolution processes are culturally and linguistically sensitive and capable of identifying, presenting, and resolving cross-cultural conflict or complaints by patients/consumers.

Standard 14. Health care organizations are encouraged to regularly make available to the public information about their progress and successful innovations in implementing the CLAS standards and to provide public notice in their communities about the availability of this information.

Office of Minority Health. (2001). *National standards for culturally and linguistically appropriate service in health care: Final report.*

This requirement has generated numerous concerns from the professional group as well as from the public. Issues were raised regarding the complexity and measurability of the outcomes as well as the overall cost for services of interpreters and translators. Health care providers are seeking guidance to seek funds to implement the standards. Others are concerned about the general nature of the standards and their limitation in providing directions for implementation and compliance. However, all health care providers are encouraged to incorporate these standards in their individual practice to ensure culturally competent and linguistically appropriate care.

To provide care that is effective, understandable, and respectful, the nurse and other health care providers need to recognize and respond to the cultural values, beliefs, and practices of the client. Culturally competent care must be provided in an environment of acceptance and respect so that the client will feel comfortable in disclosing his or her values, beliefs, and practices. This information is necessary to plan care. The nurse can explore the use of alternative or complementary healing practices, such as acupuncture or herbal and botanical remedies, and should be familiar with other traditional healing systems in planning culturally sensitive care.

Language and communication barriers must be addressed by first identifying the preferred language of the client. It must not be assumed that a client will need an interpreter solely on the basis of physical appearance or characteristics. Understanding various levels of acculturation can help the nurse in developing effective communication with the client. Some clients may be culturally assimilated and may not embrace traditional values and beliefs; some may even reject the values and beliefs of their group. It is imperative for the nurse to ensure that the recipient of health care services has a clear understanding of all information about the care and to provide opportunities to be an active participant in planning treatment options using the language the client prefers. Soliciting assistance from a community liaison, a patient advocate, or a case manager may be appropriate to establish a therapeutic bond that can enhance transcultural communication between the individual and the nurse.

DIVERSITY IN THE ORGANIZATION

Diversity in the workforce is essential in providing culturally and linguistically appropriate services. The health care organization needs to hire bicultural and bilingual staff at all levels, including staff providing direct services—such as nurses and physicians—and those in high administrative levels—such as senior executives and the board of directors, who may be affecting policies of the organization. The challenge for employers is to recruit a diverse staff that represents the population that they serve, reflecting the diversity of the community. With the current shortage of nurses in this country, we will see an increase in the number of foreign-trained nurses in the health care system. Although this situation may enhance diversity in the workforce, the new challenge will be to create a work atmosphere in which there is understanding and respect of their cultural values and beliefs. This situation may affect the working relationship of personnel within the health care system.

Organizations are directed to provide ongoing education and training in cultural competence for all health care staff at all levels and in all health care disciplines. Because cultural competence is a dynamic process, training sessions to develop cultural skills need to be ongoing and include appropriate measures to evaluate the level of cultural competence of the individual practitioner as well as the level of cultural competence of the organization. The U.S. Department of Health and Human Services recommends the following topics to be included in the training (Office of Minority Health, 2001):

- Effects of differences in the cultures of staff and patients in clinical and other workforce encounters
- Effective communications among staff and patients of different cultures and different languages, including working with interpreters
- Strategies and techniques for the resolution of racial, ethnic, or cultural conflicts between staff and patients
- Organization's written language access policies and procedures
- The applicable provisions of Title VI of the Civil Rights Act of 1964 with respect to services for individuals with limited English proficiency (LEP)
- Complaints and grievance procedures of the health care organization
- Effects of cultural differences on health promotion and disease prevention
- Impact of socioeconomic status and poverty, race, and ethnicity on access to care, service utilization, quality of care, and health outcomes
- Differences in clinical management of preventable and chronic diseases
- Effects of cultural differences among patients and staff upon health outcomes, patient satisfaction, and clinical management

LINGUISTICALLY APPROPRIATE SERVICES

Any individual who is seeking health care services and who has limited English proficiency (LEP) has the right, based on Title VI of the Civil Rights Act of 1964, to have an interpreter available to facilitate communication within the health care system. Open and clear communication is essential to develop an appropriate diagnosis and treatment. Potential errors in this area can occur when the health care provider is unable to obtain accurate information from the client with LEP. These individuals must be able to access language services, such as using an interpreter and translated materials for information necessary to understand the services and benefits available. It is important to note that some clients may not be literate even in their native language; therefore, they may not benefit from translated material that requires them to read instructions or health information. Recognizing the challenge of obtaining an interpreter 24 hours a day, the Office of Civil Rights suggests the need for the availability of interpreter services during the hours of operation. Language assistance services need to be comprehensive in that the client should receive these services from the initial point of contact with the provider, during the initial health interview, while receiving health care services, and during planning for discharge and home care. Furthermore, the health care provider must ensure that the trained interpreter follows ethical practices and guidelines. This means that strict confidentiality and privacy of information must be ensured and maintained at all times. It is the responsibility of the health care organization to ensure that the interpreters are competent and properly trained in the medical and health context. Unfortunately, use of family members or friends as interpreters is convenient and continues to be common practice in some health care settings. This practice is discouraged and can be acceptable only when the client expresses the preference to have a family member or friend be the interpreter. Clearly, there may be situations in which a formally trained interpreter is unavailable and the use of telephone interpretation is not practical; family members may then be used with permission from the client. Although telephone interpreter services are permissible, the use of a face-to-face in-person interpretation is desirable, acceptable, and appropriate.

Health care organizations are expected to make known to all their clients and families the availability of interpreter services at no cost to the client. Information about available bilingual staff can also help the client access these services. Posting translated signs in the agency that are clearly visible will be very helpful to the client. Linguistically and culturally appropriate services may be posted in community newspapers or radio stations to inform the community of the available service. To maintain the quality improvement process, the health care organizations are also encouraged to share with the public and the recipients of their services how they have implemented CLAS-related activities. An annual report may be one way to inform the public. Although these standards are directly addressed to the health care organizations, their application and relevance are clearly an expectation in professional practice.

REFERENCES

American Academy of Nursing. (1992). AAN report: Culturally competent health care. *Nursing Outlook, 40*(6), 277–283.

American Nurses Association. (1991). ANA position statement on cultural diversity: Cultural diversity in nursing practice. Council on Cultural Diversity, Congress on Nursing Practice ANA.

Campinha-Bacote, J. (1999). A model and instrument for addressing cultural competence in health care. *Journal of Nursing Education*, *38*(5), 203–207.

Campinha-Bacote, J., & Muñoz, C. (2001). A guiding framework for delivering culturally competent services in case management. *The Case Manager*, *12*, 48-52.

Cross, T. L., Bazron, B. J., Dennis, K. W., & Issacs, M. R. (1989). *Towards a culturally competent system of care: A monograph on effective services for minority children who are severely emotionally disturbed.* Washington DC: National Technical Assistance Center for Children's Mental Health, Georgetown University Child Development Center.

Dreher, M., & MacNaughton, N. (2002). Cultural competence in nursing: Foundation or fallacy? *Nursing Outlook*, *50*, 181-186.

Leininger, M., & McFarland, M. (2002). *Transcultural nursing: Concepts, theories, research and practice.* New York: McGraw Hill

Office of Civil Rights, HHS. (2000). Title VI of the Civil Rights Act of 1964: Policy guidance on the prohibition against national origin discrimination as it affects persons with limited English proficiency. *Federal Register*, *65*(169), 52762–52774.

Office of Minority Health. (2001). *National standards for culturally and linguistically appropriate services in health care: Final report.* Washington DC: Office of Minority Health.

SUGGESTED READINGS

American Nurses Association Council on Cultural Diversity in Nursing Practice. (1991). Available at: *www.nursingworld.org*.

Chin, J. L. (2000). Viewpoint on cultural competence: Culturally competent health care. *Public Health Reports*, *115*, 25–33.

Johnston, M. J. (1999). *Bioethics: A nursing perspective* (3rd ed.). Philadelphia: Harcourt Saunders. Appendix IX.

Spector, R. E. (2004). *Cultural diversity in health and illness* (6th ed.). Upper Saddle River, NJ: Prentice Hall.

CHAPTER 4

Transcultural Communication Building Blocks: Beliefs, Behavior, and Communication

KEY TERMS

- Acceptable Behavior
- Alternative Health Care System
- Biomedical Belief System
- Biomedical Health Care System
- Communication
- Folk Sector
- Holistic Belief System
- Language
- Medical Pluralism
- Mind–Body Dichotomy
- Nonverbal Communication
- Popular Health Care System
- Proxemics
- Supernatural Belief System
- Verbal Communication

OBJECTIVES

After completing this chapter, you should be able to:

- Specify the ways in which major health belief systems differ.
- Specify the ways in which major health care systems differ.
- Discuss how cultural similarities affect behavior.
- Discuss cultural diversity; in other words, describe factors other than culture that dictate how each individual within a culture behaves.

- Recognize that different cultures use different verbal communication styles.
- Recognize that different cultures use various forms of nonverbal communication.
- Accurately assess patients' verbal and nonverbal responses to pain, fear, and illness.

INTRODUCTION

Recall from Chapter 2 that transcultural communication is built, first of all, on culture. Culture, in turn, forms the basis for values. *Cultural values* (which we explore in this chapter) support the beliefs and behaviors that are accepted within each culture. Beliefs and behaviors, in turn, influence communication patterns—both verbal and nonverbal—within different cultures.

In their vital role as caregivers, nurses come into contact with people from many diverse cultures and walks of life. To provide culturally competent care, nurses must recognize and accept patients with different belief systems and styles of behavior. Moreover, nurses must be able to speak with patients who have different communication styles and who may have limited proficiency in English.

BELIEFS

As are value systems, belief systems are heavily influenced by culture. Beliefs, in turn, guide human behavior and communication. Important belief systems include religious, ethical, and political beliefs. For nurses, the cultural belief systems that govern health, illness, and health care are of greatest importance.

Different cultures have different beliefs about what causes illness, what should be done to diagnose illness, and how to treat illness. For instance, is a disease caused by a microorganism, or an evil spirit, or a disharmony in nature? Is disease most accurately diagnosed by physical assessment, by laboratory studies, or by the interpretation of dreams?

Cultural beliefs also influence how individuals within a culture define health and disease. For example, a truck driver in Los Angeles might regard a worm infestation as a sign of illness but ignore symptoms from the smog. On the other hand, a man from the island of Tristan da Cunha might acknowledge that the smog in Los Angeles makes him ill but ignore a worm infestation because it is so common on his island.

Beliefs also guide the choices people make when they seek symptom relief and the cure for illness. Will the person seek out a medical doctor (MD) or instead go to the pharmacy and purchase over-the-counter drugs? Or will the individual turn to a religious leader or a practitioner of alternative medicine? How each of us deals with disease depends upon what we believe causes disease and on who we believe is most qualified to treat disease.

Health Belief Systems

The three major types of health belief systems are

1. Biomedical

2. Supernatural

3. Holistic

The **biomedical belief system** arose from the teachings of René Descartes, a seventeenth-century philosopher. Descartes conceived of each person as a body machine. This mechanistic theory produced the concept of dualism, or the **mind–body dichotomy**; that is, the mind and body are separate from each other. According to this model, disease is caused by physiologic disturbances such as genetic disorders, biochemical imbalances, and infectious organisms. Pathologic alterations in tissues constitute evidence of disease.

As a result of their biomedical training, biomedical practitioners pay primary attention to physical complaints and pathophysiologic changes. At the same time, these practitioners deemphasize mental and emotional problems and the psychosocial component of disease. Traditional treatment usually involves administering medications or performing surgery.

Western physicians have introduced biomedicine into numerous cultures around the world. This belief system continues to dominate diagnostics and health care throughout the United States.

The **supernatural belief system**, widely accepted in traditional Hispanic, Caribbean, African, and other cultures, differs dramatically from the biomedical model. Cultural groups that believe in the supernatural model may view illness as a sign of weakness, a punishment for evil-doing, or retribution for shameful behavior such as disrespect toward elders. Some cultures also believe that illness results from the possession of the body by evil spirits or from the casting of evil spells.

Example: A 10-year-old boy from a rural Mexican family was being treated for an osteosarcoma of his distal femur. He had been transported to a medical center from a village health clinic.

According to the father, his son's cancer began when the boy was kicked by a child from a neighboring family with whom the father was feuding. The father believed that his neighbors had cast an evil spell, causing a snake to invade his son, and thus the child had developed an illness as a result of the kick. Because the father believed there was a supernatural cause for his son's illness, he also believed that the evil spell would have to be removed for the boy to be cured.

To diagnose illness, some Hispanics who have traditional values might consult with a *curandero* (healer); people in Caribbean cultures might go to a Voodoo priest or priestess. Other cultures (for example, some Native Americans) traditionally rely on dreams and divination. Traditional Native American health care providers sometimes enter a trance state to understand a person's symptoms.

In a phenomenon called **medical pluralism**, or dual use, some Native Americans turn to a medicine man to determine the true cause of an illness (i.e., why the person is out of harmony with nature) as well as to a Western physician to determine the immediate cause of the illness. Dual use or medical pluralism, is not limited to any specific cultural group. Many individuals seek and use more than one system of care.

> **Example:** A young Alaskan native woman who lived in a large city and had a regular health care provider would also return to her village for teas and herbs. She sought these remedies for a lingering condition that had not improved with biomedical treatment.

To treat illness, traditional healers who believe in the supernatural may rely on sorcery, prayer, magic, and witchcraft, using religious rites, amulets, masks, and sand painting. They may beseech their deceased ancestors or the spirit world to heal the ill person. This type of belief system also appears in the mainstream culture, despite a strong reliance on the biomedical belief system. Western Christians and Jews often turn to God when faced with life-threatening illnesses that biomedical doctors cannot cure.

The **holistic belief system** is primarily upheld by Asian cultures and some Native American cultures, although holistic beliefs have started to infiltrate traditional Western thinking. Disenchanted with the biomedical emphasis on technology, medications, and curing illness, a growing number of Americans are now interested in the concept of holistic medicine, with its emphasis on health promotion.

Unlike Western medicine, the holistic system emphasizes illness prevention and health maintenance. The major premise of this system is that there are natural laws that govern everything and every person in the universe. To be healthy, a person must remain in harmony with the natural laws and be willing to continually adjust and adapt to changes in the environment.

According to this system, illness develops when one does not properly care for the body; for example, we subject ourselves to too much cold, too much heat, too much alcohol, or an improper diet. In essence, illness results when a person fails to act in harmony with nature, causing vital elements within the body to become imbalanced. The Chinese culture refers to these elements as *yin* and *yang*; Hispanic and eastern Mediterranean cultural groups use the terms *hot* and *cold*. Too much of either of these elements (yin or yang, heat or cold) causes illness.

To restore health, the person must restore equilibrium to the body. Thus, in some cultures, people may use hot remedies if they have too much cold or cold remedies if they have too much heat. For instance, if a patient's headache is thought to be caused by a hot agent (fever, infection, diarrhea, constipation), then the person is treated with cold foods such as fresh vegetables, tropical fruits, barley, water, and cold medicines such as milk of magnesia or bicarbonate of soda.

Expressions of health problems vary from culture to culture. In some traditional and nonindustrialized countries, there are indigenous patterns of behavior referred to as "culture-bound syndromes." These are recurrent behaviors and experiences specific to a locality that fall outside Western traditional illness categories. For example, in the Filipino culture, *Amok* is an acute reaction to stress resulting in hostility and dissociative amnesia. Anorexia nervosa is typically seen in Western cultures where food is abundant, such as the United States. It is important for all health care providers to know the existence of these culture-bound syndromes.

Health Care Systems

There are four health care systems that are related to the health belief systems just described:

1. The biomedical health care system
2. The popular health care system
3. The folk or traditional health care system
4. The alternative health care system

Within the United States, many people use all of the systems, either sequentially or simultaneously.

The **biomedical health care system** combines the Western biomedical beliefs that originated with Descartes and the traditional American values of self-reliance, individualism, and aggressive action. This system is geared to conquer disease by battling the onslaught of microorganisms and diseased cells, as well as the breakdown of the body's organs due to aging. The American values of aggression, mastery over one's own fate, and dominance over nature are expressed in such phrases as "conquering disease," "winning the battle against cancer," or "beating AIDS."

The American medical system is composed of health care providers who have received specialized biomedical training and are legally and officially recognized as professionals (e.g., MDs, RNs). Licensed care providers may diagnose patients, legally prescribe and administer medications, and perform surgery. In recent years, biomedical care providers have shifted from a narrow focus on treating diseases to the broader avenues of disease prevention and health promotion.

Consistent with Western values of self-reliance and individualism, the American medical system encourages patients to learn as much as possible about their illnesses. This open information policy extends to the prognosis for a critical illness. Even when a disease may be terminal, many American physicians feel that patients have a right to know the facts about their condition and what treatment options, if any, are open to them.

Conversely, Japanese physicians are hesitant to tell patients that they have a terminal disease, preferring to keep silent, and thus sustain hope. Physicians in Bangladesh might merely suggest that terminal patients eat whatever they choose. In this way, the physician can subtly convey that the patient will probably not recover.

Teaching patients self-care is also an important component of Western medicine. For example, Western nurses routinely teach patients to give themselves insulin injections, change their own dressings, and self-administer medications. In contrast, nurses from Taiwan, where a collective orientation is more common, expect family members to actively care for the patient.

The **popular health care system**, which involves self-treatment, is the first source of care most people use, regardless of culture. For instance, the average person who has cold or flu symptoms (or who has a child with such symptoms) does not initially call a physician. Instead, the sick individual goes to the drugstore and buys a cold or flu remedy. If the remedy fails and symptoms worsen, the person may next call friends and relatives for advice on home or drugstore remedies. Only when all else fails will the person consider calling the doctor or going to a clinic.

Popular health care is also the basis for self-care groups such as Alcoholics Anonymous and various cancer support groups. Although it is often overlooked by biomedical health care professionals, popular health care provides a major source of care for a variety of problems and complaints.

The **folk sector**, or *traditional medicine sector*, includes various folk healers who use a variety of treatment modalities. Folk healers include shamans, herbalists, acupressurists, and acupuncturists. Folk healers usually maintain a holistic approach and endeavor to treat the whole person within the context of the family. Care planning and treatment take into consideration the social, physiologic, and spiritual dimensions of the patient. Folk healers are trained in their roles, and they usually have a high status in their cultural group.

Patients and their families may often move between popular, folk, and biomedical systems in various patterns of help-seeking behavior. Patients might initially select popular remedies and then shift to alternative sources of care. They may ultimately seek a biomedical practitioner only if other approaches fail. Conversely, patients may initially seek biomedical care but might then resort to folk modalities and popular treatments in light of a perceived lack of success.

Another system is the **alternative health care system**. Although they vary greatly, alternative medical practices have two common traits: (1) They differ from biomedical beliefs; and (2) they evaluate success differently from biomedical research methods.

Practitioners of alternative medicine include chiropractors, homeopaths, naturopaths, and hypnotists. Examples of alternative health care are:

1. *Diet therapy:* macrobiotics and megavitamins

2. *Mind/body control methods:* relaxation, counseling, prayer, hypnotherapy, and guided imagery

3. *Methods working with body structure and energy:* chiropractic, massage, and therapeutic touch

4. *Pharmacologic and biologic therapies:* antioxidants, oxidizing agents, and chelation therapy

Many Americans are choosing to try alternative medicine. For example, more and more patients use acupuncture as a treatment modality. This ancient Chinese healing practice is based on the concept that certain meridians in the body need to be stimulated through puncturing to reestablish body equilibrium and restore health. According to a national survey published in *The Landmark Report on Public Perceptions of Alternative Care* (Landmark, 1998), 42% of the 1500 adults interviewed had used some form of alternative care during 1996 and 1997. Of these individuals

- 74% had used alternative care *in addition* to traditional care.

- 15% had *replaced* traditional care with alternative care.

- 11% had used alternative care along with *and* as a replacement for traditional care.

Respondents were also asked how important the *availability* of alternative care was for them when choosing a health plan. Of the respondents

- 31% felt that alternative care was *very important* when choosing a health plan.

- 36% felt that alternative care was *somewhat important* when choosing a health plan.

- 33% felt that alternative care was *not important* when choosing a health plan.

Finally, researchers attempted to forecast the outlook for alternative care by asking respondents if they had experienced any *change of opinion* toward alternative care over the past five years. Of the respondents

- 40% stated that their opinion toward alternative care had grown *more positive.*

- 58% stated that their opinion of alternative care had *not changed.*

- 2% stated that their opinion of alternative care had become *more negative.*

BEHAVIOR

Cultural values dictate human behavior to a vast extent. Culture encourages each of us to think, feel, and then act in certain prescribed ways—thus the reason for cultural similarities. On the other hand, each culture is made up of individuals whose beliefs and behavior reflect some aspects of their culture, but not all aspects—thus the reason for cultural diversity.

Cultural Similarities

Culture encourages us to behave in a way similar to others in our culture while behaving quite differently from people of other cultures. Indeed, people are consciously or subconsciously rewarded for being with and acting like people who resemble themselves.

Example: Most middle-class Americans are culturally conditioned to eat three meals a day, work five days a week, and celebrate certain holidays at specific times of the year according to definite traditions (Christmas, Easter, July 4th, Thanksgiving). But persons from other cultures—especially from Asia and Africa—have vastly different eating, working, and celebrating habits, and they may view traditional Western activities with skepticism.

Culture dictates what is **acceptable behavior** when sick. Identifying what is acceptable behavior within your patient's culture will help you understand your patient's reactions to illness. In some cultures (e.g., Asian and Native American cultures), patients are expected to be stoic and silent when in pain. On the other hand, within the Mediterranean culture, it is acceptable to express pain with loud complaints and dramatic gestures.

Culture also influences whether a person is willing to talk about symptoms or emotions with care providers. For instance, Asian cultures typically value a subtle approach to problems and the restraint of strong feelings. Thus, Asian patients may find it difficult to speak openly with strangers about symptoms or emotional problems. Conversely, middle-class white Americans, raised in a society that values open expression, may welcome an opportunity to frankly discuss their symptoms with health care providers.

As do larger cultures, subcultures foster similar behavior patterns among members. These behavior patterns are based on specific subcultural values and beliefs. Traditionally, nurses have proudly worn white uniforms, as well as the caps and pins that represent their particular school of nursing. Furthermore, the nursing profession has its own organizations and educational programs that clarify nursing goals and behaviors and clearly set nursing apart from other professional health care subcultures such as physicians' assistants.

Hospitalized patients also form a subculture. Patients are expected to conform to hospital policies, wear hospital garb, eat hospital food at designated times, take their medications as prescribed, and undergo laboratory tests when convenient for hospital personnel—often as early as 5:30 AM. Furthermore, patients are asked to cheerfully endure invasions of their privacy for the sake of their health. People who enter a hospital for treatment must put aside their usual roles (mother, businessman, teacher) and behave as a patient within the hospital subculture.

Cultural Diversity

Although each culture dictates general values and behavior among its members, factors other than culture dictate how each individual within that culture should behave. Important factors that influence behavior patterns and habits include:

1. Age
2. Gender

3. Length of residence in the United States

4. Rural or urban residence

5. Occupation

6. Level of education

7. Use of English

8. Degree of acculturation

9. Socioeconomic class

10. Personality characteristics

11. Previous experiences

12. Personal beliefs

13. Religious beliefs

14. Sexual orientation

Example: Suppose you were asked to predict what a typical middle-class white American would have for dinner. Your chances of predicting the meal accurately would be better if you knew the person's age (is the person a teenager who loves junk food?), socioeconomic status (is steak too expensive?), religion (is pork permitted?), personal experiences (does the person identify a home-cooked chicken dinner with a happy home life?), and personal beliefs (is the person a vegetarian?). So many individual factors other than culture play a role in selecting a meal that it is impossible to know the menu for a typical American dinner.

Likewise, when caring for patients from different cultures, remember that culture provides only the broad canvas of information upon which each person paints the details of his or her personality and life experiences. Even if you are an expert on a patient's culture, you will not be able to predict exactly how that person is going to behave when ill. The person's educational level, presence or lack of support systems, degree of medical knowledge, past experiences with illness and hospitalization, and many other factors will ultimately determine how that individual will respond to illness.

COMMUNICATION CONSIDERATIONS

Remember to recognize the individuality of each patient, regardless of culture.

COMMUNICATION

At its most basic level, **communication** occurs when a person (the sender or encoder) sends a message to another person (the receiver or decoder). The message may be **verbal** (spoken or written in a language) or **nonverbal** (conveyed through facial expressions and body language). Communication is most effective when the message received is exactly the same as the message that was sent and both sender and receiver agree on the meaning of the message.

Communication fails when (1) the sender's message is blocked for some reason and the receiver never gets the message; or (2) the message is distorted. Distortion occurs when the message has a different meaning for the receiver than the sender intended. Distortion is amplified when the sender and receiver fail to seek feedback and clarify the message. Factors that can distort messages include anger, fatigue, fear, pain, and anxiety.

Moreover, communication may be blocked when senders and receivers come from different cultural, ethnic, racial, socioeconomic, or educational backgrounds. For example, Japanese Americans with a traditional background may not want to question or challenge health care providers, especially physicians. As a result, some Japanese American patients may silently accept a physician's recommendations even when they do not understand the reasons for the medications or procedures that are ordered.

Verbal Communication

Verbal communication, which includes both the spoken and written word, depends upon language. **Language** is the code senders use to carry their messages.

> **COMMUNICATION CONSIDERATIONS**
>
> Language allows us to initially identify, label, attach significance to, and evaluate our experiences.

Language barriers can create severe communication problems between senders and receivers. Language barriers may arise from the use of different language systems (e.g., the sender is speaking English and the receiver is speaking Spanish), or they can arise when the sender uses technical terms, abbreviations, idioms, or regionalisms that are unfamiliar to the receiver (e.g., when a nurse uses medical terms when explaining a procedure to a layperson).

Every culture has *standards* for verbal communication—especially for word choice, the degree of emotion considered appropriate, volume and speed of speech, inflection, directness, and the use of silence.

Word Choice. American speech is filled with abbreviated words, slang, and jargon. Americans tend to communicate in an informal way with superiors and subordinates alike. In contrast, the Japanese use of language is distinguished by many levels of formality and degrees of politeness, depending upon the status of the people who are conversing. The Japanese also make distinctions between men's and women's speech. Thus, the choice of words for the Japanese depends largely on the relationship between the people who are communicating. An expression such as "What is this?" can be said in several different ways, depending on the sender's relationship to the receiver.

Emotional Expressiveness, Tone, Pitch, Volume of Voice, and Speed of Speech. Traditionally, black and white American cultures differ in the amount of expressiveness allowed when verbally communicating. For example, white American middle-class culture values a controlled tone of voice and some emotional restraint. On the other hand, many black Americans are more verbal and value emotional expressiveness in a conversation or discussion. Because of this difference in values, middle-class whites may not understand that blacks tend to express themselves dynamically and, thus, may misinterpret their loud voice volume as aggression (Glanville, 2003).

However, even whites vary in the emotion and expression in their voices. For instance, Appalachians characteristically speak very slowly, and they seem to dwell on each word, giving their speech a hesitant, disjointed quality. Unlike blacks and whites, many Asians and Native Americans display great emotional restraint in their speech patterns, speaking slowly and quietly. These cultures may value the ability to endure pain and grief with silent stoicism.

In marked contrast, southern Europeans are typically warm, expressive, and sometimes dramatic in both their verbal and nonverbal communication. Generally, they are not stoic about pain but will loudly express their discomfort. People from more expressive cultures may view Asians and Native Americans as withdrawn, shy, and silent.

Voice Inflection. When one person talks to another, the emphasis that is placed on certain words often says more than the words themselves. For example, "What do you *need* now?" sends a different message from "What do you need *now*?" In many languages, the inflection given to the syllables of some words can change the meaning.

Directness in Speech. Some cultures value politeness more than others. Americans, being members of an impatient and future-oriented culture, like to get to the point of a conversation rather than wasting time on lengthy preliminaries or long silences. Americans may be quite direct when communicating with others. Mexicans, on the other hand, strive to be polite, diplomatic, and tactful. They may take the time for small talk and then lead into a discussion.

Use of Silence. Some cultures value silence, whereas other cultural groups feel that silence is a vacuum that must immediately be filled with words. Among some Native Americans, silence is an essential element of showing respect and understanding. In some Arab cultures, silence may indicate concern for personal privacy. The French, Spanish, and Eastern European cultures interpret silence as a sign of agreement. Silence during a conversation also gives each person an opportunity to speak without having to interrupt.

Nonverbal Communication

Experts estimate that as much as two-thirds of all communication is nonverbal, consisting of messages that are conveyed from one person to another via body language and facial expressions. Specific forms of nonverbal communication throughout the world include the examples that follow.

Gestures and Facial Expressions. The world's many cultures differ vastly in their interpretation of some gestures and facial expressions, whereas the interpretation of other gestures is fairly standard. For example, in nearly all cultures, people use their mouths and eyebrows to convey surprise, anger, pleasure, and fear, and they use hand gestures to convey openness or intimidation. The same words that may be "read" as an insult if the speaker is glaring might be understood to be teasing if the speaker is smiling. Common types of nonverbal communication may differ in meaning from culture to culture. For example, a smile may imply acceptance and compliance, but for other cultural groups, a smile may simply mean respect and social grace.

Eye Movement and Eye Contact. There is an old saying that "the eyes are the windows of the soul." Because the eyes are thought to reveal a person's true nature, many Americans assume that it is a negative sign when a person avoids eye contact. It is not unusual to hear an American say, "Look at me when I talk to you," or "She must be lying. Did you notice that she avoided looking at us?" American nurses and physicians usually note if a patient avoids eye contact when they perform a psychosocial assessment.

Other cultures view the significance of eye contact differently. Some Asians and Native Americans believe that prolonged eye contact is rude and an invasion of privacy. Native Americans may divert their eyes to the floor when they are paying attention or thinking. Muslim women may avoid eye contact as a show of modesty. Appalachians tend to avoid eye contact because they feel that it expresses hostility and aggressiveness. In India, the amount of eye contact that is appropriate depends on one's social position (people of different socioeconomic classes avoid eye contact with each other).

COMMUNICATION CONSIDERATIONS

In Western cultures, prolonged eye contact may be considered a sign of intimacy, especially in conjunction with the use of touch. Nurses need to guard against prolonged eye contact with patients when performing invasive procedures.

Use of Personal and Interpersonal Space (Proxemics). The amount of personal space that people need as a comfort zone varies from individual to individual and from culture to culture. For Western culture, research has identified the following four zones of interpersonal space (Giger & Davidhizar, 2003):

1. *Intimate space:* from contact to 18 inches. This space is normally reserved for people who are in close relationships. Nurses frequently occupy this space as they bathe and feed patients.

2. *Personal space:* from 18 inches to 4 feet. This space is commonly used for interaction between friends. It is also useful for patient counseling.

3. *Social space:* from 4 to 12 feet. The business of everyday life is most often conducted within social space.

4. *Public space:* greater than 12 feet. This space is used during lectures and speeches.

Typically, middle-class Americans, Canadians, and the British feel uncomfortable when forced to stand or sit close to people they do not know well. In fact, white Americans who feel that their personal space is being violated may react with anger and withdrawal. Other cultures welcome physical closeness. Latin Americans, Africans, black Americans, Indonesians, Arabs, and the French prefer to stand close to one another when holding a conversation.

Problems can arise when, for example, a North American from a British background speaks with a Latin American. The North American, feeling that his personal space is being violated, may find himself backing away from his Latin American acquaintance. The Latin American may interpret the North American's reaction as a sign of aloofness, dislike, or unwillingness to talk. In reality, the problem is not one of personalities, but of proxemics.

Touch. Depending on whether it is gentle, sensual, harsh, or brutal, touch conveys many meanings. We use touch to connect with others and establish feelings of warmth, approval, emotional support, and intimacy. On the other hand, touch can communicate anger, aggression, frustration, and a desire to control others by invading their personal space. Touch (or a laying on of hands) may also be regarded as therapeutic.

Cultures have specific guidelines for times and situations when it is acceptable to touch others. Middle-class Americans typically consummate a business deal with a handshake; some Native Americans, however, view a firm handshake as aggressive and even offensive. Many Westerners think nothing of kissing or hugging a friend as a form of greeting when meeting in public places. In traditional Asian cultures, such behavior is reserved for intimate relationships in private settings.

Posture. Posture helps to communicate how one person feels toward another. For instance, middle-class Americans may lean in the direction of individuals that they like or respect. Posture can also communicate a tense or relaxed state. Crossed arms tend to distance the parties in an interaction, whereas greeting someone with open arms suggests a desire to be close to that person. Rigid muscles and a flexed body may indicate physical pain.

COMMUNICATION CONSIDERATIONS

Be aware of the patient's verbal and nonverbal communications as well as inconsistencies between them.

The message conveyed by nonverbal communication may be far closer to the truth than verbal communication. For example, the man who pounds on the table and shouts "I'm not angry!" is clearly showing his anger. The preoperative patient who looks worried and tense but tells you she is not afraid of surgery is showing her fear through her expressions and body language.

You also need to observe for communication that is *vocal but still nonverbal*. This universal type of communication includes moaning, sighing, gasping, crying, laughing, and coughing.

Assessing Verbal and Nonverbal Responses

The various communication styles that arise from cultural differences can make it difficult for nurses to accurately assess their patients' verbal and nonverbal responses to illness or surgery. Evaluating patients' responses to pain can be particularly challenging.

> **Example:** Karen Green, a young RN, was having a hectic night on a postoperative floor. During her rounds, she stopped to check on Mrs. Wong, a middle-aged Chinese woman who had been in the United States for five years and who spoke limited English. Mrs. Wong had undergone knee surgery that morning. Karen asked Mrs. Wong if she needed anything for pain. Mrs. Wong, although she seemed restless and unable to sleep, shook her head and said "No."
>
> Next, Karen took Mrs. Wong's vital signs and found that her blood pressure and pulse were elevated and her respirations were rapid and shallow. Karen also noted that Mrs. Wong's face looked tense and drawn and that she resisted attempts to help her move or turn.
>
> Mrs. Wong's roommate, Mrs. Tortano, was a middle-aged Italian American woman who had spent her entire life in her city's Italian community. Mrs. Tortano, who had had surgery on her shoulder that morning, was clutching Karen's hand and shouting, "Nurse, nurse, give me a shot! I can't stand the pain!" Karen noted that Mrs. Tortano's blood pressure and pulse were elevated and her respirations were rapid. When asked to move or breathe deeply, Mrs. Tortano vigorously shook her head, "No!"

Even though each woman expressed her discomfort differently, Karen concluded that both of her patients were experiencing severe pain that required medication. The fact that pain can evoke such different verbal and nonverbal responses may be due to personality or cultural differences or both.

Karen had learned that Asian cultures value a more stoic response to pain, whereas the Italian culture tolerates a more emotive response to pain. Karen also recognized that individuals do not necessarily conform to the communication style accepted in their culture. Thus, some Asians may be more emotive, and some Italians more stoic when dealing with pain, grief, and other difficult circumstances.

> **•••• COMMUNICATION CONSIDERATIONS ••••**
>
> Patients from different cultures may communicate their pain, anxiety, fear, and other powerful feelings and emotions in different ways. Thus, nurses need to carefully assess their patients in order to accurately decode their transcultural communication—both verbal and nonverbal.

Techniques for eliciting assessment data from patients from different cultures is discussed in detail in Chapter 11.

REFERENCES

Giger, J. N., & Davidhizar, R. E. (2003). *Transcultural nursing: Assessment and intervention* (4th ed.). St. Louis: Mosby.

Glanville, C. L. (2003). People of African American heritage. In L. D. Purnell & B. J. Paulanka, *Transcultural health care: A culturally competent approach* (2nd ed.). Philadelphia: Davis.

Landmark Healthcare. (1998). *The Landmark report on public perceptions of alternative care.* Sacramento, CA: Landmark Healthcare.

SUGGESTED READINGS

Alternative medicine: Separating fact from fiction. (1994). *The University of Texas Lifetime Health Letter, 6*(5), 1, 6.

Andrews, M. M., & Boyle, J. S. (2002). *Transcultural concepts in nursing care* (4th ed.). Philadelphia: Lippincott.

Avery, C. (1991). Native American medicine: Traditional healing. *Journal of the American Medical Association, 265*(17), 2271–2273.

Axtell, R. E. (Ed.). (1993). *Do's and taboos around the world* (3rd ed.). New York: Wiley.

Dossey, B. M., & Dossey, L. (1998). Attending to holistic care. *American Journal of Nursing, 98*(8), 35–38.

Keegan, L. (1998). Getting comfortable with alternative and complementary therapies. *Nursing 98, 28*(4), 50–53.

Lapierre, E. D., & Padgett, J. (1991). How can we become more aware of culturally specific body language and use this awareness therapeutically? *Journal of Psychosocial Nursing, 29*(11), 38–41.

Matsumoto, D. (1989). Face, culture, and judgments of anger and fear: Do the eyes have it? *Journal of Nonverbal Behavior, 13*, 171–188.

Meadows, J. L. (1991). *Multicultural communication* (pp. 31–42). Binghamton, NY: The Hawthorne Press.

Purnell, L. D., & Paulanka, B. J. (2003). *Transcultural health care: A culturally competent approach* (2nd ed.). Philadelphia: Davis.

Spector, R. E. (2004). *Cultural diversity in health and illness* (6th ed.). Upper Saddle River, NJ: Pearson Prentice Hall.

Sue, D. W., & Sue, D. (1990). *Counseling the culturally different: Theory and practice* (2nd ed.). New York: Wiley.

CHAPTER 5

Transcultural Communication
Stumbling Blocks

KEY TERMS

- Barrier
- Bias
- Cultural Blind Spot Syndrome
- Dialect
- Ethnocentrism
- Idiom

- Nursing Ritual
- Racism
- Regionalism
- Simultaneous Dual Ethnocentrism
- Stereotype

OBJECTIVES

After completing this chapter, you should be able to:

- Identify barriers to effective transcultural communication between patients and nurses.
- Describe the process by which people from diverse cultures go from fearing each other to liking each other.
- Identify and describe the three types of racism that are found in our society.
- Define ethnocentrism and explain how this barrier blocks transcultural communication.
- Describe the different types of language barriers that can impede transcultural communication.

- Develop an awareness of the various dialects, regionalisms, and idioms that distinguish the speech of people from different races, ethnic groups, and regions.

- Identify ways in which differing perceptions and expectations can complicate communications between nurses and patients from diverse cultures.

INTRODUCTION

Communication between nurses and patients from different cultures is often complicated by different values, beliefs, traditions, expectations, and languages. As you work with patients from multicultural backgrounds, you will find that these differences raise barriers to transcultural communication. This chapter discusses communication barriers in terms of their underlying dynamics, and their impact on nurses, patients, and nursing care. Chapter 9 describes practical strategies for overcoming transcultural communication barriers in the health care arena.

BARRIERS TO TRANSCULTURAL COMMUNICATION

There are eight important **barriers** to transcultural communication in nursing: (1) lack of knowledge, (2) fear and distrust, (3) racism, (4) bias and ethnocentrism, (5) stereotyping, (6) ritualistic behavior, (7) language barriers, and (8) differences in perceptions and expectations.

Lack of Knowledge

The failure to understand cultural differences in values, behaviors, and communication styles is a common stumbling block for nurses who work in transcultural settings. Nurses who are not knowledgeable about cultural differences risk misinterpreting patients' attempts to communicate. As a result, patients may not receive the proper care.

Remember that each culture dictates what is "normal" behavior when sick. For example, Japanese patients might react with silent obedience to your requests; white middle-class patients might wish to discuss their nursing care with you; Italian patients might dramatically express their discomfort; and an inner city youth might loudly demand your attention. Nurses who are unaware of cultural differences may mistakenly expect all patients to communicate in the same way, regardless of culture.

Furthermore, nurses who have not learned about which behaviors are acceptable in different cultures may attribute a patient's behavior (e.g., silence, withdrawal) to the wrong reason or cause, resulting in faulty assessment and intervention.

Example: A nurse was teaching a prenatal class to a group of white, Hispanic, and black adolescents. The nurse used some words that Bonita, a Hispanic teenager, did not understand. Bonita asked the nurse to explain what the words meant. The nurse, who wanted to cover the rest of her lesson, told Bonita that she would talk with her about the words after class. But when class was over, Bonita abruptly left the room.

The nurse, who was not knowledgeable about Hispanic culture, incorrectly assumed that Bonita either had forgotten that she was to remain after class or had decided that she had more important things to do.

Had the nurse known more about the culture and behavioral patterns of Hispanics, she would have realized that:

- Hispanics typically view nurses and teachers as authority figures and expect them to initiate actions. Thus, Bonita expected the nurse to call her name and remind her to stay after class.

- Many Hispanic children receive a great deal of close supervision and attention from adults. Bonita might have felt that she should not have been made to wait until after class to receive answers to her questions.

- Hispanic children are raised to be respectful and quiet. Bonita overcame her shyness when she asked the nurse a question. If the nurse had known more about the behavioral patterns of Hispanic children, she would have invited Bonita to ask her questions again at the end of class. Because Bonita did not receive a cue from the nurse that it was all right to speak, she assumed it would be rude to raise her hand.

Thus, this nurse-instructor incorrectly attributed Bonita's behavior to forgetfulness or disrespect. Because the nurse did not understand the culturally based reasons for Bonita's behavior, she missed a valuable opportunity to expand Bonita's grasp of prenatal care.

Fear and Distrust

Fear, dislike, and distrust are emotions that all too often erupt when people from diverse cultures first meet. Rothenburger (1990) has identified seven stages of adjustment that individuals pass through during their initial encounters with people of different cultures that they do not know or understand. These stages are:

1. *Fear:* When first meeting someone from a different culture, many people feel threatened. Each person perceives the other person as different and, therefore, dangerous. Usually, as people become better acquainted with each other, the fear gradually dissipates, only to be replaced by dislike.

2. *Dislike:* Dislike is a much milder emotion than fear. Group members have a tendency to dislike people who behave or communicate differently from what is considered "the norm" in that culture or group. For example, a working-class black person might dislike a middle-class white person because white people tend to be less vocal and expressive than many black people, and thus appear insincere and weak.

3. *Distrust:* People from different cultures are often suspicious of each others' actions and motives because they lack information. For example, a white nurse who does not realize the importance of family in Vietnam may be suspicious of the new Vietnamese nurse who allows family members to participate in a patient's care instead of providing all of the care herself. Unfortunately, unless there is pressure to change their attitudes, some people never do progress beyond fear, dislike, and distrust to the next stage of acceptance.

4. *Acceptance:* Usually, if two people from different cultures share enough good experiences over a period of time, they will begin to accept each other rather than resent each other.

5. *Respect:* If individuals from diverse cultures are open minded, they will allow themselves to see and admire qualities in one another. For example, a Japanese nurse who has been trained to defer to authority might admire the white American nurse who challenges authority. Acceptance and admiration, in turn, foster respect.

6. *Trust:* Once people from diverse cultures have spent enough quality time together, they usually are able to trust each other. For example, a white American nurse will eventually trust the foreign-born nurse who consistently provides good patient care and finishes assignments on time. Once people trust each other, they may finally learn to genuinely like each other.

7. *Like:* For people to like each other, they must share many things in common. To reach this final stage, individuals from diverse cultures

must be able to concentrate on the human qualities that bind people together, rather than the differences that pull people apart.

This evolution of a relationship from fear to trust has been dramatized in films. For instance *The Defiant Ones*, starring Tony Curtis and Sidney Poitier, is the story of two escaped convicts—one white and one black—who are chained together. At first, the two men dislike and distrust each other. However, the men are forced to work together in order to survive. By the time the film ends, the men have established a mutual trust and respect.

Racism

Racism in American nursing is a formidable barrier that strangles transcultural communication between nurses and patients and between nurses and other health care providers. Because nursing is regarded as a "caring profession," nurses find it difficult to acknowledge that racism exists in the health care workplace. Indeed, for most Euro-American nurses, discussions of racism in American nursing are taboo (Barbee, 1993).

Barbee's article points out that there are three types of racism:

1. *Individual racism:* Individuals are discriminated against because of their visible biological characteristics; for example, black skin or the epicanthic fold of the eyelid in Asians.

2. *Cultural racism:* An individual or institution claims that its cultural heritage is superior to that of other individuals or institutions. For example, during World War II, the Nazis claimed that their Aryan genetic and cultural heritage was superior to the Jewish heritage. They justified persecution of the Jews by convincing themselves that the Jews were an inferior people.

3. *Institutional racism:* Institutions (universities, businesses, hospitals, schools of nursing) manipulate or tolerate policies that unfairly restrict the opportunities of certain races, cultures, or groups. For example, at one time, black nurses were not allowed to join the American Nurses Association (ANA). This policy prevented black nurses from having a voice in the regulation of nursing practice and policies.

Because nurses perceive themselves as individuals who regard all people as equal, most nurses (black and white) will talk about *cultural diversity* but avoid the word *racism*. Nevertheless, racism exists. For example, in a classic study by Morgan in 1984, researchers found that Euro-American nursing students perceived black patients more favorably than did black people, and they perceived Euro-American patients as more favorable than any other group.

At the institutional level, white students have been admitted more readily to schools of nursing than black students. Racism is also a factor in the low enrollment numbers of black students in baccalaureate nursing programs compared with two-year programs. Within the workforce, black nurses have complained about not being promoted as readily as white nurses (see Chapter 15). Also, black nurses have had difficulty publishing in Euro-American nursing journals.

Racism will undermine the nursing profession for as long as nurses deny its existence and refuse to talk about it openly and honestly. In the words of Barbee (1993):

> One of the flaws in the profession is an unwillingness to recognize that racism is endemic in nursing and health care. This unwillingness results in a lack of discussion about racism and leads to responses that exacerbate the problem.

Bias and Ethnocentrism

Whatever their cultural background, people have a tendency to be **biased** toward their own cultural values and to feel that their values are *right* and the values of others are *wrong* or *not as good*. Many people are surprised to discover that the values and actions they so admire in their own culture may be looked upon with suspicion by people from other cultures, who are equally biased.

COMMUNICATION CONSIDERATIONS

The belief that one's own culture or traditions are better than those of other cultures is called **ethnocentrism**. The person who is ethnocentric tends to antagonize and alienate people from other cultures.

Simultaneous dual ethnocentrism is a component of every nurse–patient relationship. Nurses are assessing, judging, evaluating, and reacting to patients on the basis of their own cultural values, medicocentric points of view, and expectations. Simultaneously, patients are using their cultural values to judge and evaluate their nurses and the Western health care system. As DeSantis (1994) pointed out:

> The concept of a simultaneous dual ethnocentrism makes nurses keenly aware that they, their patients, their colleagues, and everyone

else in the clinical setting are operating under the influence of personal cultural rules, some of which are shared and some of which are not.

Attitudes toward Western medicine constitute one of the biggest barriers to transcultural communication between American nurses and patients. American nurses tend to be heavily biased toward the Western biomedical health care system because most of them have been educated in this system. Indeed, many nurses feel that the biomedical system is the best (and even the only) approach to patient care. They may view other health belief systems with suspicion and even contempt, refusing to acknowledge that another approach might have some merit. This ethnocentric attitude can alienate patients from other cultures, who fully believe that *their* therapeutic interventions also have merit. Here is an example of how simultaneous dual ethnocentrism can severely damage the nurse–patient relationship.

Example: Juan Perez, a Mexican immigrant, was hospitalized with a fever of unknown origin. A major conflict developed between the head nurse and Mr. Perez's family when the family insisted that a *curandero*, or folk healer, visit the patient. When the curandero appeared on the ward with various healing paraphernalia, the head nurse demanded that the healer leave the patient's room at once. The nurse's attitude so upset Mr. Perez that his family signed him out of the hospital against medical advice. Had the nurse been willing to at least acknowledge Mr. Perez's health care beliefs, he would have been more willing to accept her biomedical beliefs.

When white American nurses care for people from other cultures, they may be biased not only toward their own health care system but also toward other learned values, such as cleanliness.

Example: During a clinic visit, a Caucasian nurse assessed that a Native American child had severe impetigo. The nurse observed that the child appeared dirty and that the mother had not thoroughly washed her hands. The nurse concluded that because the child was dirty, the mother was not taking adequate care of her child.

The nurse's assessment was based on a value she learned while studying nursing: that is, that cleanliness is essential and basic to good health. Her observations translated into a value judgment based on Western bias: "Cleanliness is good. Therefore, a good mother always keeps her child clean."

The mother perceived correctly from the nurse's demeanor and tone of voice that this authority figure from the dominant white culture disapproved of her and her parenting skills. She also suspected that the nurse was planning to impose her expectations concerning cleanliness and childrearing.

The Native American mother found herself nodding yes but tuning out the disapproving nurse's instructions. The young mother would have been much more inclined to listen had the nurse been sensitive in her approach rather than dictatorial. The nurse could have said: "I'm sure that you've noticed that your baby has a problem with his skin. When did the problem start? What have you done thus far for the itching? Has it helped? Let's think about this problem together and see what we can do."

By admitting and overcoming her own rigid bias toward cleanliness, the nurse would have conveyed that the child needed attention without appearing to judge the mother's standard of cleanliness or her child care skills. As a result, the mother would have been more inclined to listen to the nurse and follow through on her suggestions.

> **• • • • COMMUNICATION CONSIDERATIONS • • • •**
>
> Cultural biases can distort your perception of other people's values and behavior and thus damage your ability to communicate. To overcome your biases, you must first acknowledge that they exist.

Stereotyping

A cultural **stereotype** is the unsubstantiated assumption that all people of a certain racial and ethnic group are alike. For example: *All Eskimos are reserved, deliberate, and noncommittal.* Certainly, some or even the majority of Eskimos may be reserved, deliberate, and noncommittal, but it is cultural stereotyping to state that all Eskimos have these traits. Stereotyping is particularly destructive when negative traits or characteristics are imposed on all members of a cultural group. For example: *All Native Americans are at risk for alcoholism.*

Although you must avoid negatively stereotyping patients from different cultural groups, it is nevertheless important to learn about the representative characteristics of different groups. This knowledge will help to smooth and ease your interactions with patients from other cultures.

For example, if you know that Eskimos are raised to be reserved and noncommittal, you will not be offended when Eskimo patients respond to your assessment questions with silence or monosyllables. Conversely, if you are aware that Italian patients tend to be more flamboyant as a group, you will not be surprised when your Italian patients respond to their problems with dramatic gestures and tears.

COMMUNICATION CONSIDERATIONS

To avoid stereotyping, remember that patients are individuals with unique experiences and thus may not conform to many (or any) of the characteristics ascribed to their cultural group. Thus, some Eskimos may be outgoing, and some Italians may be reserved.

Cultural blind spot syndrome is a form of stereotyping that is a problem for many nurses and physicians. Cultural blind spot syndrome is the belief that "Just because the client looks and behaves much the way you do, you assume that there are no cultural differences or potential barriers to care" (Buchwald, Caralis, & Gany, 1994). For example, white American nurses may assume that white American patients believe in the same cultural values as they do. This assumption is false. As you learned in Chapter 2, white Americans come from many different ethnocultural backgrounds—Irish, Russian, German, Jewish, and English to name but a few. In addition, white nurses and patients may also belong to different subcultures that have different values. For example, a white male patient of Italian descent who is gay will probably have somewhat different values than a white Irish American male nurse who is married and has three children. The negative impact of cultural blind spot syndrome on patient care is discussed further in Chapter 11.

Ritualistic Behavior

A ritual is a set procedure for performing a task. In the past, students in nurse's training were taught to perform their duties in a ritualistic manner. Even today, **nursing rituals** persist. Many nursing rituals are beneficial, such as always performing certain safety checks when preparing and administering medications. However, other rituals, such as always excluding family from the bedside during treatments, are unnecessary and may upset patients and their families. Unfortunately, many nurses are so in the habit of performing certain rituals that they become deeply disturbed when these rituals are challenged.

> ● ● ● **COMMUNICATION CONSIDERATIONS** ● ● ●
>
> As you care for patients, ask yourself which nursing rituals are really necessary and which rituals are outdated. If there is no scientific or logical reason to follow a ritual, try to create a new routine that will benefit you and your patient.

Language Barriers

Language provides the tools (words) that allow people to express their thoughts and feelings. Thus, language barriers present a grave threat to transcultural communication between nurses and patients. There are several types of language barriers that impede communication in the United States. These barriers include:

1. Foreign languages
2. Different dialects and regionalisms
3. Idioms, slang, and "street talk"

Foreign Languages, Dialects, and Regionalisms. Even when nurses and patients speak the same language, misunderstandings can arise. But when patients come from countries or households where English is *not* the native tongue, the resulting language barrier can bring communication to a halt, producing frustration and conflict.

Unfortunately, it is not possible to be familiar with the hundreds of languages and dialects spoken by patients from different countries and cultures. As noted in Chapter 1, over 6000 languages and dialects are spoken today. In addition, the number of people in the United States (all potential patients) who speak languages other than English is growing.

According to the 2000 census, individuals who spoke languages other than English constituted approximately 13.8% of the population. According to a U.S. Education Department report on languages during the 1980s, the number of Spanish speakers increased 65%, and speakers of Asian languages rose 98%. Spanish was the most frequently spoken language at home. In some states, the percentage of persons speaking another language is higher than the national norm (U.S. Bureau of Census, 2001B).

Large communities of people who speak languages other than English are flourishing in southern California, Texas, New Mexico, and Arizona. In Los Angeles alone, over 100 languages other than English are spoken. These languages range from the familiar Spanish tongue to the more exotic language of Gujarati, which is spoken in western India (Compton's, 1995). Moreover, there are many more communities throughout the country where different languages and traditions are common.

As if coping with people who speak different languages is not enough, nurses must also be aware that there are hundreds of dialects and regionalisms. Webster's Dictionary defines a **dialect** as the distinctive way a language is spoken or written in a given locality or by a given group of individuals. A **regionalism** is a word, phrase, pronunciation, or custom peculiar to a given region. For example:

- There are three major Chinese dialects: Mandarin, Cantonese, and Shanghainese.

- There are 600 Filipino languages and dialects, of which the most common are Tagalog, Ilocano, Ilonggo, and Cebuano.

- Spanish is not divided into dialects, but there are some regional differences in the use of particular words and phrases. The most recent influx of migrant workers in California speak Mextec, not Spanish.

- Ebonics, or African American English, was first discussed in 1975 in *Ebonics: The True Language of Black Folks*, a book by psychology professor Robert L. Williams. Williams derived the word *ebonics* from *ebony* (for black) and *phonics* for "the scientific study of speech sounds." Williams pointed out that black people are often accused of using bad English when actually they are speaking their own language or dialect, which is based on standard English. In December of 1996, the Oakland School Board in California officially recognized ebonics as a language or dialect. Concerned that the majority of black students who spoke ebonics were not doing well in school, the board passed a resolution calling for improved instruction in standard English (Barnhart & Metcalf, 1997).

To communicate effectively with patients who are not proficient in English, you will need an interpreter. A skilled interpreter can help you, your patient, and your patient's family overcome the anxiety and frustration produced by language barriers. Chapter 10 describes methods for communicating with patients with limited English proficiency, both with and without an interpreter.

Idioms, Slang, and Street Talk. Sometimes the language barrier—and the type of interpreter needed—may not fit the conventional mold just discussed. For example, if you are from a white middle-class background, you may find yourself at a loss to understand the characteristic terms, **idioms**, or expressions used by patients from English-speaking subcultures, be they ghetto blacks, Appalachian hillfolk, or teenagers fluent only in the latest street slang. For example, a nursing student from an upper-class background failed to understand the adolescent girls in a clinic until another nurse explained that *poppers, fizzers,* and *wa-was* referred to prescribed medicines.

Black American speech is particularly rich in idioms. In her book *Black Talk: Words and Phrases from the Hood to the Amen Corner*, Geneva Smitherman-Donaldson (1994) explains that the word *hood* means the neighborhood where a person has grown up and feels comfortable. The phrase *amen corner* refers to the corner in a traditional black church where the older church members (usually women) sit. These women, regarded as the *watchdogs of Christ* lead the congregation in amens.

Some black expressions that you may hear as you work with some black patients in neighborhood clinics or hospitals have the following meanings (Smitherman-Donaldson, 1994):

- *Bad* means excellent or good.
- *BMT* means black man talking. This term is used to express authority.
- *Can't kill nothing and won't nothing die* means having a difficult time.
- *Get on the good foot* means to correct what needs improving.
- *Git out my face* means stop confronting me.
- *Glass house* is a drug house.
- *Come out of a bag* means to behave differently than expected.
- *Hoodoo man* is a person skilled in voodoo.
- *The Nation* refers to the Nation of Islam, a black Muslim group.
- *Soul* means the essence of life, passion, or emotion.

Different Perceptions and Expectations

When people from different cultures try to communicate, their best efforts may be thwarted by misunderstandings and even serious conflicts. In health care situations, misunderstandings often arise when the nurse and patient have different perceptions and expectations and consequently misinterpret each others' messages.

Misunderstandings due to cultural differences commonly arise in situations involving food and drink. Imagine that you are taking care of a postoperative Vietnamese female patient who, as her culture dictates, is almost constantly attended by her family. You want to clearly instruct family members that they are not to give the patient anything to drink. Because the family speaks only Vietnamese, you motion that the patient is not to drink, and you explain through an interpreter that the patient must not drink.

When you return from your lunch break, you find your patient vomiting, and you observe an empty bowl of soup on her table. Obviously, the family ignored your instructions and fed the patient soup. If you angrily say "I told you not to give her anything to drink!" your reaction will be that of many nurses in this situation.

However, you later learn from the interpreter that the family knew that they should not give the patient water, but they assumed that broth would be beneficial. Vietnamese believe that the sick need to drink broth to rebuild energy. Your intended message (do not drink anything) was not understood by the patient's family, and you failed to grasp the family's perception of your instructions (broth is not water, and therefore all right to drink). As a result, the patient's family gave her broth and you became frustrated.

COMMUNICATION CONSIDERATIONS

When there are cultural, behavioral, and language differences between nurses, patients, and patients' families, there is a greater probability that patients will misunderstand nursing care instructions. To prevent conflicts and misunderstandings, make sure that the message you send the patient is the same message that the patient receives. When there is a language barrier, you will need to work closely with an interpreter.

Another common area of conflict between nurses and patients from diverse cultures involves the perception of health promotion and disease prevention. For example, Hispanics—whose culture is based on honor and pride—may be taught from childhood to bravely accept illness and pain as an inevitable part of human existence. For this reason, traditional Hispanics may see no reason to submit to mammograms or vaccinations (Sabatino, 1993). In the words of the former Surgeon General Antonia Novello:

> Hispanics are fatalistic. We've been taught that you live, you suffer, you die. That's the way life is. The idea has never been presented that if you take care of your health, if you go to the doctor early, you won't have to suffer pain or discomfort.

Expectations that patients have of nurses and physicians may also lead to transcultural communication problems. For example, Japanese patients generally look to their family members for the majority of their care, rather than to nurses. Even physicians are not in charge; instead they are thought of as *skilled and sympathetic technicians* whose job it is to help families cure the patient (Rothenburger, 1990). Nurses or physicians need to recognize the importance of the Japanese patient's family as caregivers and to always communicate with the family before making any important decisions concerning the patient's care.

REFERENCES

Barbee, E. L. (1993). Racism in U.S. nursing. *Medical Anthropology Quarterly, 7*(4), 346–362.

Barnhart, D. K., & Metcalf, A. (1997). *America in so many words: Words that have shaped America.* Boston: Houghton Mifflin.

Buchwald, D., Caralis, P. V., & Gany, F. (1994). Caring for patients in a multicultural society. *Patient Care, 28*(11), 105–123.

Compton's Interactive Encyclopedia. Copyright © 1994, 1995, 1996, Compton's NewMedia, Inc.

DeSantis, L. (1994). Making anthropology clinically relevant to nursing care. *Journal of Advanced Nursing, 20*(4), 707–715.

Gannett Service. (1994, January 19). Many don't use English at home. *San Antonio Express News.* ISA.

Morgan, B. S. (1984). A semantic differential measure of attitudes toward black American patients. *Research in Nursing and Health, 7*, 155–172.

Rothenburger, R. L. (1990). Transcultural nursing: Overcoming obstacles to effective communication. *AORN Journal, 51*(5), 1349–1363.

Sabatino, F. (1993). Culture shock: Are U.S. hospitals ready? *Hospitals, 67*(1), 22–25, 28–31.

Smitherman-Donaldson, G. (1994). *Black talk: Words and phrases from the hood to the amen corner.* Boston: Houghton Mifflin.

Williams, R. L. (1975). *Ebonics: The true language of black folks.* St. Louis: Institute of Black Studies. (This book was based on papers submitted by Robert L. Williams in 1973.)

SUGGESTED READINGS

Campinha-Bacote, J. (1995). The quest for cultural competence in nursing care. *Nursing Forum, 30*(4), 19–25.

Cochran, M. M. (1998). Tears have no color: The medical world is not always prepared for the collision of cultures. *American Journal of Nursing, 98*(6), 53.

Cravener, P. (1992). Establishing therapeutic alliance across cultural barriers. *Journal of Psychosocial Nursing, 30*(12), 10–14.

Fairlie, A. (1992). Nurse-patient communication barriers. *Senior Nurse, 12*(3), 40–43,

Fielo, S. B., & Degazon, C. E. (1997). When cultures collide: Decision making in a multicultural environment. *Nursing and Health Care Perspectives, 18*(5), 238–243.

Foong, A. (1992). Challenging the tower of Babel: The increasing diversity in cultures. *Nursing, 5*(5), 12–25.

Giger, J. N., & Davidhizar, R. E. (Eds.). (2003). *Transcultural nursing: Assessment and intervention* (4th ed.). St. Louis: Mosby.

Malone, B. L. (1993). Caring for culturally diverse racial groups: An administrative matter. *Nursing Administration Quarterly, 17*(2), 21–29.

Mattson, S., & Johnson, L. (1992). Integration of cultural content into a psychiatric nursing course to change students' attitudes and decrease anxiety. *Nurse Educator, 17*(4), 5.

Newman, J. (1998). Managing cultural diversity: The art of communication. *Radiographic Technology, 69*(3), 231–246, 249.

Purnell, L. D., & Paulanka, B. J. (2003). Purnell's model for cultural competence. In L. D. Purnell & B. J. Paulanka (Eds.), *Transcultural health care: A culturally competent approach* (2nd ed.). Philadelphia: Davis.

Sherer, J. L. (1993). Crossing cultures: Hospitals begin breaking down the barriers to care. *Hospitals, 67*(1), 22–25, 28–31.

Thiederman, S. B. (1986). Ethnocentrism: A barrier to effective health care. *Nurse Practitioner, 11*(8), 52–59.

Tips for overcoming cultural barriers. (1998). *Same-Day Surgery, 22*(4), Supplement 4.

Trossman, S. (1998). Diversity: A continuing challenge. *American Nurse, 30*(1), 1, 24–25.

Urden, L. D., Stacy, K. M., & Lough, M. E. (2001). *Thelan's critical care nursing: Diagnosis and management* (4th ed.). St. Louis: Mosby.

CHAPTER 6

Transcultural Communication within the Health Care Subculture

KEY TERMS

- Commercial Subculture
- Nursing Subculture
- Patient Subculture
- Professional Subculture
- Professional Values

- Vulnerable Stranger
- Western Biomedical Ethnocentrism
- Western Biomedical Perspective

OBJECTIVES

After completing this chapter, you should be able to:

- Discuss cultural values, beliefs, and behaviors of the Western health care system.
- Describe potential communication conflicts among health care providers, management, and patients within the hospital environment.
- Describe the nursing subculture and its development.
- Discuss the perspective of the patient in the hospital environment.
- Identify three strategies to help you recognize and deal with Western health care ethnocentrism in the hospital setting.

INTRODUCTION

Learning about culture requires learning about yourself. It is often easier and more interesting to learn about cultural beliefs and practices that are exotic or different from your own. However, to develop a true appreciation for the power of culture, it is necessary to learn about how our own culture affects our beliefs, our actions, and our expectations. This knowledge is imperative in the profession of nursing, in which there are multiple layers and overlaps in a variety of cultural and subcultural groups. Understanding these layers and overlapping loyalties and beliefs will help you identify communication problems and illuminate potential solutions.

This chapter explores the concept of transcultural communication within the subculture of the Western health care system. It explores the overlapping subcultures within the health care system and identifies specific areas in which miscommunications can occur because of cultural differences. By understanding the perspectives of professional, business, and patient subcultures, nurses working within their professional nursing subculture will learn how to broker communications within and among these varied groups.

WESTERN HEALTH CARE SYSTEM SUBCULTURE

The Western health care system includes all individuals and organizations involved in the education, professional practice, delivery, business, and consumption of health care in what is called Western culture. The Western health care system is a subculture of white Western culture. The Western health care system is a reflection of the culture and society in which it belongs. The white Western culture and its tradition promotes an almost exclusive belief in and reliance on the biomedical belief system.

Members of this tradition value *technology* almost exclusively in the struggle to conquer disease. Western health care professionals gather enormous amounts of data (laboratory tests, invasive procedures, x-rays, body scans, review of systems) in order to diagnosis and treat the underlying pathophysiology. Their goal is to rapidly resolve the patient's symptoms with biomedical interventions and ultimately cure the pathology. Although some elements of the popular and traditional, or folk, sectors of health care have gained credence within Western health care (including the recent recognition of a variety of alternative or complementary health practices), the dominant belief system remains biomedical.

The strong, shared belief in the biomedical approach to health care has sometimes resulted in **Western biomedical ethnocentrism**, a serious barrier to communication. This ethnocentrism is displayed in the derision that greets patient use of or provider interest in alternative health practices. Even the term *alternative* indicates that these practices are outside the accepted biomedical practices and thus will be tolerated only if they do not interfere with the *real* biomedical treatment plan. Interest in alternative (more recently called *complementary*) therapies has increased, particularly for patients with cancer, AIDS, chronic pain, stress, and psychological disorders. Research on these remedies has been funded by the National Institutes of Health. Nevertheless, patients and providers who are interested in, use, or practice these therapies may find it difficult to communicate with providers who work within the strongly biomedical culture of Western health care.

• • • • COMMUNICATION CONSIDERATIONS • • • •

The strong biomedical culture of the Western health care system may result in communication problems between providers and patients who choose to use alternative or complementary therapies.

Although the Western health care system is a subculture of its own, it is also a multifaceted collection of other identifiable subcultural groups. The goals of diagnosis and treatment using biomedical methods are shared in varying degrees in the specialized health care settings of private physician or nurse practitioner offices, hospitals, clinics, home care, rehabilitation, and long-term care facilities. The goals change somewhat in long-term care facilities and hospice, yet they are still strongly connected with the Western health care system values, beliefs, and behaviors.

The hospital is the most visible and well known of the subcultural settings of Western health care, owing in large part to the use of hospital settings in popular television programs. The hospital setting is a microcosm of the Western health care system and an excellent place to explore the issues of transcultural communication within Western health care.

HOSPITAL SUBCULTURE

The hospital in Western culture is a complex organization dedicated to the common goal of health care delivery. *Health* is generally understood to be the absence, minimization, or control of disease processes. The hospital is a complex organization with multiple players involved in a variety of hierarchical relationships founded on the goal of health care delivery. The various players in the organization may work in concert or in conflict, depending on the cultural expectations that they bring to this environment.

PROFESSIONAL SUBCULTURE

One of the major subcultures operating within the hospital is the **professional subculture** of the direct care providers. This professional subculture includes nurses, physicians, therapists, and pharmacists. These practitioners are licensed by legislative authority to provide health care. Although each of these professional groups has a strong subgroup identity and subculture, they share in the professional health care values of beneficence and nonmalfeasance (being of benefit and doing no harm) established in the Hippocratic oath.

Professional groups have codes of conduct that define appropriate behavior, including veracity (telling the truth), fidelity (loyalty and keeping promises), and professional and patient confidentiality. Western health care professionals also embrace the value of individual autonomy, which is a major part of white Western culture as discussed in Chapter 2.

> **•••• COMMUNICATION CONSIDERATIONS ••••**
>
> The practice of informed consent and patient rights is based on the value of individual autonomy. The Patient's Bill of Rights is prominently displayed in Western hospitals.

Members of the professional subculture in the Western hospital setting strongly support the value of being a benefit to patients, and they have been educated to put the patient first, largely without regard to the financial costs or effective use of resources. Professionals focus on their relationships with individual patients and the accurate biomedical diagnosis and treatment. They have taken an oath and are licensed to help patients and this oath and the licensing requirements guide their behaviors and communications.

COMMERCIAL, OR BUSINESS, SUBCULTURE

The **commercial** (or business) **subculture** is another strong subculture in Western hospitals. As complex organizations, hospitals need expert business managers and administrators who can maintain an environment for meeting the goal of delivering health care. The values that members of the business subculture bring to the hospital environment include maintaining the health of the organization through support systems (supplies, building maintenance), financial responsibility (paying employees, collecting payments), and market competition. The language of *fiscal responsibility, the bottom line, outcomes-based care*, and the increasingly popular *managed care* provides external evidence of the business culture in health care.

COMMUNICATION PROBLEMS BETWEEN SUBCULTURES

All hospitals need competent and dedicated administrators and managers from the business culture to provide the environment for health care delivery. All hospitals also need competent and dedicated care providers from the professional subculture. When these cultures clash, communication conflicts result, producing disagreements about cost-effective care. Professional care providers tend to focus on effective care based on the biomedical belief system: Is the pathology corrected or mitigated? Managers and administrators ask difficult questions about the monetary value or worth of a treatment and the cost–benefit analysis of the health outcome. Discussions that argue these points are strongly based in the cultural beliefs of the participants.

Bringing cost into a treatment decision is strongly counter to the professional cultural ethic. For example, to eliminate mild or moderate chest pain, physicians may advocate coronary artery bypass surgery for single-vessel heart disease as the best option, even though surgery is more expensive than other interventions. Ignoring the costs of treatments is strongly counter to the responsible business ethic. From a business perspective, a cost–benefit analysis of surgery versus the less expensive medical management is central to making a treatment decision. Knowing that there are professional and administrative cultural issues involved in discussions helps all parties reach better compromises and solutions (McArthur & Moore, 1997).

OTHER HEALTH CARE SUBCULTURES

There are other important subcultures in Western health care related to and yet significantly different from the hospital subculture. These subcultures include the areas of long-term care and community-based health care. Although these subcultures are affiliated with the hospital, they have their own guiding values and beliefs. Communication problems may arise when professionals from these subcultures interact with hospital-based professionals. For example, the long-term care subculture encompasses a wider range of *successful outcomes* than the control of pathophysiology of disease processes and includes expected progressive decline and death. Patients are called residents to reflect the combination of home and health care environments. Professionals who move from the acute-care to the long-term care environment frequently experience a culture shock as they learn new behaviors and expectations for professional care.

Community-based health care environments include a wide variety of settings: for example, hospice, home-care, public health clinics, ambulatory care, and school health. Each of these settings combines Western health care values with the values that guide the particular setting.

THE PROFESSIONAL NURSING SUBCULTURE

Nursing is the largest professional group in hospital health care. As members of the hospital subculture, nurses are directly involved in the cultural communication conflicts described. Numerous sources (Campinha-Bacote, 2003; Leininger, 2002; Martin & Nakayama, 2004; Spector, 2004) have emphasized the importance of effective intercultural communication and cultural competence in the practice of nursing and other health care professions. Nurses have their own distinct professional nursing subculture, a culture started by Florence Nightingale and the other founders of professional nursing.

Studying the Nursing Subculture

The beliefs, values, and behaviors common to nurses today—the **nursing subculture**—can be traced to the development of nursing as a profession by Nightingale. Nurses first learn this culture in nursing school. Nursing students have varying degrees of exposure to the culture of nursing before entering nursing school through personal experience, family history, or viewing nurses in media presentations.

The organizing belief system used in my basic nursing program was the statement: Nursing is the *bio-psycho-socio-spiritual* care of the patient. As nursing students, we learned the pathophysiology of disease, then the psychological and social aspects of disease, and finally the need to find appropriate spiritual guidance for patients. The order of these aspects of holistic nursing practice was not accidental, and it reflects the dominance of the Western biomedical view of health care.

As students, nurses study the American Nurses Association Code for Professional Nurses, which outlines the appropriate beliefs and behaviors for nurses. From their nursing professors, course assignments, and state Nursing Practice Act they learn the activities of nursing. In this way, the culture of nursing—the common values, beliefs, and practices—is learned, shared, and transmitted from one generation of nurses to the next.

In the 1960s, 1970s, and 1980s, Marlene Kramer and her colleagues studied the *culture shock* experienced by baccalaureate nursing graduates when they entered the hospital nursing environment (for example, see

Kramer, 1968, 1970, 1974; Lewandowski & Kramer, 1980). These researchers promoted the concept of *biculturalism* for new graduate nurses, meaning that they needed to retain their *high idealism* learned in nursing school, while learning to deal with the *daily practicalities* of the hospital nursing work environment. This research, an explicit recognition of the culture of nursing, pointed out the variation between that culture in school and in the hospital.

Practicing within the Nursing Subculture

Although specific behaviors may differ from hospital to hospital, nurses who form the hospital nursing subculture share many values, beliefs, behaviors, and rituals, such as the traditional shift report. The hospital nursing subculture in turn overlaps, has commonalties with, and also conflicts with the hospital subculture, the professional subculture, and the dominant American culture. Nurses in long-term care and community-based health care environments have similar overlaps and conflicts.

The use of technology is a major part of the hospital nursing environment, with higher status attributed to those nurses who work in the high-technology environments of intensive care and emergency departments. It is no accident that these are the environments that are portrayed on popular television programs; they reflect the Western cultural value of conquering or mastering the biomedical disease enemy—preferably using state-of-the-art technology.

The nursing subculture also shares the professional ethic of beneficence and a relative dislike for or distrust of the concern with the costs or business side of patient care. This attitude can result in difficult and frustrating communications with managers and administrators. Nurses must learn the language and values of both of these hospital subcultures.

Leininger (2002) has included descriptions of the culture of nursing in her book on transcultural nursing. She describes transcultural nursing as using "a comparative view to know and understand the meaning of cultures and care within specific environmental and holistic contexts." Leininger advocates a thorough understanding of the nursing culture in order to provide the best nursing care possible and claims that, in essence, all health care interactions are transcultural (Leininger, 2002).

Leininger's discussion of the core features of the culture of nursing captures important developments, such as the change from nurses as handmaids of physicians (a feature of the early era of nursing, 1945 to 1975) to nurses as collaborators with multiple care professionals in more autonomous roles (post-1975). Leininger also points out that within this culture, nurses value self-care and self-reliance; for example, they expect patients to actively participate in their own care. These values may create problems when American nurses care for patients or work with nurses from cultures that believe that others (e.g., the family) should care for the patient. Nurses need to be aware of their professional and personal biases when dealing with patients and other nurses.

Nursing Subculture and Language

Nursing is defined as a culture because it is learned in nursing schools, shared among multiple health care environments, and transmitted from one generation of nurses to the next. Nurses follow rules of behavior that are both specific to a particular health care environment and generalized to the profession of nursing. Whether defined as a culture or a subculture, nursing has a distinct identity, value system, and expected behaviors (Suominen, Kovasin, & Ketoca, 1997). One of these expected behaviors is *language*.

Nurses use professional biomedical language on the job and readily converse with other health care professionals in terms often incomprehensible to people not employed in health care. Some of this language is shared by all health care professionals: for example, terms relating to pathophysiology, diagnostic tests, and treatments. Other language is specific to particular environments (e.g., the operating room), where personnel use special terms that can be incomprehensible to health care providers from other areas. Although the specialty-specific dialects may cause minor communication problems between care providers, these problems may become major for patients and their families who struggle to understand. The language of Western health care is English, which can add to communication problems with nonnative English health care workers (see Chapter 15).

> **Example:** This problem is reflected in my experience with a specialty dialect when I first worked on a cardiac medical–surgical unit. The first day I listened to morning report, I heard about the patient who was a "cabbage times three"—which I later learned referred to the patient with a three-vessel coronary bypass graft (or *CABGx3* in the surgical notes). This dialect was not covered in my nursing education or in my hospital orientation, and I can only wonder what non-health care workers would make of being described as a "cabbage times three!"

THE PATIENT SUBCULTURE

As mentioned in Chapter 2, patients in hospitals also form a distinct subculture. Whatever their culture of origin, professional or occupational subculture, adopted cultural identity, degree of assimilation or acculturation to Western culture, or religious identity, patients all become members of a distinct **patient subculture** when treated in the hospital setting.

Because the language of health care is unique and the schedules of daily activities are new, every patient enters this hospital environment as a **vulnerable stranger** in need of care (Toumishey, 1989). Repeated treatment in hospitals produces some patients who become more or less acculturated to the hospital culture. However, even these patients remain vulnerable with each hospital admission, because when patients enter the hospital they become isolated from their usual life routines.

> **Example:** On being ordered to take his clothes off for examination, a newly admitted patient explained this revelation:
>
> > This incident, trivial in itself, brought two points home to me in immediate succession. To start with, my own individuality, my own independence, my private self and what it meant to me, had, as though by her telling remark, been taken away from me. Until a couple of hours ago, outside the hospital environment, I had been a free agent, free in so far as it is possible to choose, free to determine, and free to exercise my own will on matters large and small. But in the hospital I felt entrapped. I had entered a new environment, a new culture, which had its own established rules and norms. I was now expected to learn and follow the rules of the new culture—in other words play the role of patient (Laungani, 1992, p. 10).
>
> This patient, a psychology professor who had conducted research in many hospital environments, now found himself a stranger in the health care environment.

Laungani describes his three-month hospitalization and how he had to learn to survive in this relatively familiar (to him) culture in a new and unfamiliar role. He emphasizes how patients are expected to be compliant and grateful. He also discusses how the nature of being dependent and vulnerable interplays with learning how to behave as a good patient and fit in so that he could get the help he so desperately needed. Toumishey (1989) describes how vulnerable strangers (such as Professor Laungani) must determine an appropriate new role, the accepted meanings of behavior in the new environment, expectations of others, and methods of coping. This task is difficult enough for patients who are familiar with the Western health care culture, as Professor Laungani certainly was. It is far more difficult for those unfamiliar with it or from a radically different cultural background.

When patients become *residents* in long-term care facilities, they face additional challenges. Now the subculture encourages a *homelike* environment, yet this is frequently overshadowed by the needs of the community of residents. "Home" is no longer an individual personal space, a primary value in Western culture, but a shared living space (frequently intimately shared) with continued and increasing dependency on caregivers for daily needs. Caregivers and residents become a close community/family with extended relationships, which may be enjoyable or difficult and may continue day after day. In addition, the personal cultures of the caregivers may radically conflict with those of the residents.

NURSES AS CULTURE BROKERS BETWEEN SUBCULTURES

Nurses work within and through all of these Western health care subcultures. Nurses need to be aware of their own subculture as well as the values and associated behaviors of the other subcultures to be effective in holistic patient care delivery and patient advocacy.

In order to participate effectively in transcultural communications in the hospital environment, you need to evaluate your own beliefs, biases, and behaviors. Self-assessment exercises help with this evaluation. In addition to these, study your work environment from the perspective of culture. What are the rituals that you observe and participate in? What are the patterns of movement, daily routines, clothing, equipment, and language that are essential elements of your work? These elements express the cultural values of the **Western biomedical perspective**: efficiency, timeliness, technology, and science/pathophysiology. You will continue to be a part of this culture of health care, but you will be sensitized to the wider meaning of your beliefs and actions.

Try to see your work environment as a stranger (patient) would. One method of doing this is to experience the role of the stranger. Visit an environment where you do not know the language or accepted behaviors. Attend a public event in a neighborhood where you are in the minority. Attend a religious service of which you have no previous knowledge or experience. Any of these experiences will help you understand the feeling of being a stranger.

Observe yourself and your colleagues for signs of ethnocentric reactions—shock, anger, laughter—when confronted with beliefs and behaviors that conflict with the world view of Western biomedicine. Although surprise may be a common part of contact with different health care beliefs and practices, as a professional you need to demonstrate respect. As discussed in other parts of this book, a successful transcultural communication requires that health care professionals show respect for and work with patients to understand their health care needs and beliefs. Remember that your own biomedical belief system may seem odd or silly to the patient. To work toward a successful and mutually acceptable negotiated treatment plan, explore how your Western beliefs fit or conflict with the patient's beliefs.

Brokering between Patients and the Health Care Subculture

Nurses are in a vital position for negotiating between the patient culture and the Western health care culture. There are three steps basic to this brokering:

1. Be aware of the fact that the Western health care system is a culture of its own with rituals and language often incomprehensible to patients.

2. Carefully explore the patient's cultural background and needs.

3. Explore and explain the particular patient subculture to which the patient has been admitted.

An awareness of the potential confusion and conflicts among these three subcultures is necessary for nurses to function as both patient advocate and professional health care provider. Nurses can effectively translate the complexities of health care to patients, as well as translate the patient's values and beliefs to other Western health care providers.

Brokering between Professional Subcultures

Nurses must work with a variety of personnel in Western health care and can become proficient in communicating in a variety of situations. For example, nurses faced with explaining the use of alternative (complementary) therapies to colleagues in the Western biomedical system would be wise to explore these therapies in an open and interested manner. It is also important to share research on the use and success of the therapies with colleagues in a nonthreatening manner. The standard research approach for testing the efficacy of therapeutic touch provides an excellent example. There are a number of articles on the use of therapeutic touch in a variety of nursing settings (Daley, 1997; Easter, 1997; Fryback & Reinert, 1997; Kotora, 1997; Snyder, 1997). When selecting references to share with Western practitioner colleagues, include articles from the more mainstream and accepted biomedical perspective as well as newer, alternative publications.

Nurses skeptical of alternative health care practices should familiarize themselves with this literature because patients often use a variety of alternative (complementary) treatments.

> **•••• COMMUNICATION CONSIDERATIONS ••••**
>
> Understanding the various subcultural groups in Western health care is the first step in effective communications. Exploring these groups and their interactions and conflicts will increase effectiveness as a health care provider. Learning how to translate and broker communications among the various groups will help avoid the frustrations of miscommunications and potential problems.

REFERENCES

Campinha-Bacote. (2003). *The process of cultural competence in the delivery of health care services* (4th ed.). Cincinnati, OH: Transcultural Care Associates.

Daley, B. (1997). Therapeutic touch, nursing practice and contemporary cutaneous wound healing research. *Journal of Advanced Nursing, 25*(6), 1123–1132.

Easter, A. (1997). The state of research on the effects of therapeutic touch. *Journal of Holistic Nursing, 15*(2),158–175.

Fryback, P. B., & Reinert, B. R. (1997). Alternative therapies and control for health in cancer and AIDS. *Clinical Nurse Specialist, 11*(2), 64–69.

Kotora, J. (1997). Therapeutic touch can augment traditional therapies. In M. T. Knobf & C. T. Donovan (Eds.), Practice corner. Practice tips from the Yale Cancer Center, New Haven, CT. *Oncology Nursing Forum, 24*(8), 1329–1330.

Kramer, M. (1968). Role models, role conceptions, and role deprivation. *Nursing Research, 17*(2), 115–120.

Kramer, M. (1970). Role conceptions of baccalaureate nurses and success in hospital nursing. *Nursing Research, 19*(5), 428–439.

Kramer, M. (1974). *Reality shock: Why nurses leave nursing.* St. Louis: Mosby.

Laungani, P. (1992). *It shouldn't happen to a patient.* London: Whiting & Birch.

Leininger, M. (2002). *Transcultural nursing: Concepts, theories, research & practices* (3rd ed.). New York: McGraw Hill.

Lewandowski, L. A., & Kramer, M. (1980). Role transformation of special care unit nurses: A comparative study. *Nursing Research, 29*(3), 170–179.

Martin, J., & Nakayama, J. (2004). *Intercultural communication in contests* (3rd ed.). New York: McGraw Hill.

McArthur, J. H., & Moore, F. D. (1997). The two cultures and the health care revolution. *Journal of the American Medical Association, 277*(12), 985–989.

Snyder, J. R. (1997). Complementary therapies in hospice care. Therapeutic touch and the terminally ill: Healing power through the hands. *American Journal of Hospice and Palliative Care, 14*(2), 83–87.

Souminen, T., Kovasin, M., & Ketoca, O. (1997). Nursing culture—some viewpoints. *Journal of Advanced Nursing, 25*(1), 186–190.

Spector, R. E. (2004). *Cultural diversity in health and illness* (6th ed.). Upper Saddle River, NJ: Prentice Hall.

Toumishey, L. H. (1989). Strangers among strangers: Clients and health practitioners in health care settings. *Nurse Education Today, 9*(6), 363–367.

SUGGESTED READINGS

Gropper, R. (1996). *Culture and the clinical encounter: An intercultural sensitizer for the health professions.* Yarmouth, ME: Intercultural Press.

Leininger, M. (1997). Transcultural nursing research to transform nursing education and practice: 40 years. *Image: Journal of Nursing Scholarship, 29*(4), 341–347.

Lipson, J., Dibble, S., & Minarik, P. (1996). *Culture & nursing care: A pocket guide.* San Francisco: UCSF Nursing Press.

UNIT ONE
EVALUATION

EVALUATING YOUR TRANSCULTURAL COMMUNICATION GOALS AND BASIC KNOWLEDGE

The following exercises highlight some of the concepts that we discussed in this unit. Make a note if you are selecting a different option than you would have *before* studying Unit One.

Exercise One: Altering Transcultural Communication Approaches

After reading the chapters in Unit One, answer these questions as honestly as possible.

1. What are your major transcultural communication goals?
   _____
   _____
   _____
   _____

2. What factors in *yourself might support* your goals?
   a. _____
   b. _____
   c. _____

3. What factors in your *clinical setting might support* your goals?
   a. _____
   b. _____
   c. _____

4. What factors in *yourself might hinder* your goals?
   a. _____
   b. _____
   c. _____

5. What factors in your *clinical setting might hinder* your goals?
   a. _____
   b. _____
   c. _____

6. In what ways would you like to alter or improve your transcultural communication style or approach?

_____

_____

Exercise Two: Reviewing Your Transcultural Interaction Diary

1. Have you had any positive interactions with patients from other races or cultures? _____

   What did you learn about each patient's cultural values and beliefs?

   _____

   _____

   What communication style (verbal and nonverbal) did each patient use?

   _____

   _____

   How did you respond to each patient's communication style?

   _____

   _____

2. Have you had any *difficult or unsuccessful* interactions with patients from other cultures?

   _____

   _____

   Which transcultural communication *stumbling block* do you feel was instrumental in creating a negative interaction?

   _____

   _____

   Are you aware of any other stumbling blocks such as bias, stereotyping, or ritualistic behavior that could damage your transcultural interactions?

   _____

   _____

3. Chapter 6, "Transcultural Communication within the Health Care Subculture," suggests that you visit an environment where you do not know the language or social customs. How did you feel about this experience?

   _____

   _____

   What did you learn from this experience that you can apply to your work with people from other cultures?

   _____

   _____

Exercise Three: Evaluating Your Readiness for Unit Two, Developing Your Transcultural Communication Skills

Write a brief response to these questions, which are drawn from topics discussed in Chapters 1 through 6.

1. What is the objective of communication in nursing?

   _____

   _____

2. What is communication competence?

   _____

   _____

   On a scale from 1 to 10 (10 being the most competent), how competently do you communicate with patients from other cultures?

   _____

   _____

3. Give four reasons why it is currently so important for nurses to learn transcultural communication skills.

   a. _____
   b. _____
   c. _____
   d. _____

4. Cultural values are principles or standards that members of a cultural group share in common. Values serve at least seven important functions:

   a. _____
   b. _____
   c. _____
   d. _____
   e. _____
   f. _____
   g. _____

   What cultural values do you believe in?

   _____

   What subcultures do you belong to?

   _____

   What subcultural values do you believe in?

   _____

5. What are the three major health belief systems?

   a. _____

   b. _____

   c. _____

   Do you accept the health beliefs of patients who are from other cultures?

   _____

   Why or why not? _____

   _____

6. What are the four major health care systems?

   a. _____

   b. _____

   c. _____

   d. _____

   What experiences have you had with each health care system?

   _____

   _____

7. What factors determine a person's response to illness?

   _____

   _____

   _____

   What do you feel is acceptable behavior for a hospitalized patient?

   _____

   _____

8. Each culture has different standards for *verbal* communication. Give transcultural examples of the following:

   a. Word choice: _____

   b. Emotional expressiveness and volume: _____

   c. Voice inflection: _____

   d. Directness: _____

   e. Use of silence: _____

9. *Nonverbal communication* also differs from culture to culture. Give examples of different types of nonverbal communication.

   a. _____

   b. _____

   c. _____

   d. _____

   e. _____

10. According to Rothenburger, what are the seven stages that people pass through during their initial encounters with individuals from different cultures?

   a. _____

   b. _____

   c. _____

   d. _____

   e. _____

   f. _____

   g. _____

   What stages have you experienced when developing relationships with people from other cultures?

   _____

   _____

11. What is simultaneous dual ethnocentrism, and how does it affect every nurse–patient relationship?

   _____

   _____

12. In what ways do language barriers present a grave threat to communication between nurses and patients?

   _____

   _____

   What different types of language barriers have you encountered in the clinical area?

   _____

   _____

   _____

13. What are the four different types of transcultural conflicts that can occur within the health care subculture? Give an example of each.

   a. _____

   b. _____

   c. _____

   d. _____

   What types of transcultural conflicts have you experienced in the clinical area?

   _____

   _____

UNIT TWO

Developing Transcultural Communication Skills

UNIT TWO
ASSESSMENT

ASSESSING YOUR TRANSCULTURAL COMMUNICATION SKILLS

Exercise One: Assessing How Comfortable You Feel When Communicating with Patients from Other Cultures

As you communicate with people from other cultures, you will gradually become more comfortable during transcultural interactions. The more comfortable you feel, the more comfortable your patients will feel. Exercise One will help you assess your current level of comfort with transcultural interactions. The statements that follow contain assignments that you might receive in the clinical area or community. Using the following five levels of comfort, rate how you feel about performing each assignment.

- Level 1: I feel very uncomfortable.
- Level 2: I feel rather uncomfortable.
- Level 3: I feel fairly comfortable.
- Level 4: I feel comfortable.
- Level 5: I feel very comfortable.

1. *Assignment:* Go into a market in an ethnic neighborhood and ask the store personnel about the different foods that are available and how to prepare them. **1 2 3 4 5**

2. *Assignment:* Go to an ethnic pharmacy and speak with the pharmacist about which over-the-counter drugs the people in the neighborhood tend to purchase. **1 2 3 4 5**

3. *Assignment:* Visit a cuandero or folk healer and learn about the various healing modalities that he or she uses. **1 2 3 4 5**

4. *Assignment:* Admit an older Asian female patient who is accompanied by many concerned, attentive family members. **1 2 3 4 5**

5. *Assignment:* Admit an Italian patient who is constantly crying and grabbing onto your hand. **1 2 3 4 5**

6. *Assignment:* Provide home care to a 4-month-old child whose mother has placed open scissors (resembling a cross) under the child's pillow in order to ward off evil spirits.   **1 2 3 4 5**

7. *Assignment:* Give a complete bath to a Vietnamese woman with the husband and older children present throughout the procedure.

    1 2 3 4 5

8. *Assignment:* Have a medical interpreter help you collect verbal data from a patient who does not speak English.   **1 2 3 4 5**

9. *Assignment:* Admit a patient who does not speak English without the help of an interpreter.   **1 2 3 4 5**

Exercise Two: Assessing Your Point of View toward Transcultural Nursing Situations

What is your attitude toward transcultural nursing situations? Do you feel that it is very important to consider the patient's cultural background when giving care? Or do you feel that cultural considerations are much less important than other aspects of nursing care? Select the one answer that best describes your point of view *now*, before you proceed with the chapters in this unit. There is no scoring for these questions.

1. The nurse in the nurse–patient interaction needs to
    a. elicit the patient's perspective about being ill
    b. share food with the patient
    c. adopt the patient's customs
    d. efficiently manage the care of the patient

2. A culturally sensitive nurse
    a. is knowledgeable about cultural traits
    b. adheres to institutional regulations
    c. adapts communication style to be congruent with the patient's expectations
    d. develops expertise in asking questions to gather patient data

3. The attention that should be allotted to communication in transcultural settings is
    a. little or none because few instances are truly cultural exchanges
    b. fairly significant because many patients are from diverse cultural backgrounds
    c. of consequence in only some settings
    d. extremely important and necessary for holistic nursing care

4. When working with a patient in the emergency room who has limited English proficiency, I would
   a. have a close family member interpret for the patient
   b. rely on a telephone language service for pertinent information
   c. make an effort to find a qualified interpreter
   d. attempt to communicate with the patient using a phrase chart

5. When interacting with patients, I would
   a. encourage them to express their views of illness
   b. discourage personal beliefs, because they have little connection to the health care plan
   c. elicit information about their family
   d. insist that they need to comply with their care plan for their own good

Exercise Three: Using Your *Transcultural Interaction Diary*

1. In Unit One you set up your *Transcultural Interaction Diary*. To help you apply the principles that you will learn in Unit Two, record any positive or negative transcultural transactions that involve (a) acting as a participant-observer in an ethnic community, (b) establishing communication with a patient from another culture; (c) overcoming transcultural communication barriers, and (d) working with and without an interpreter.

2. You may want to write some of your diary entries in the form of a *process recording*. A process recording (or a verbatim report) is a written record in which you record every word that you and the patient exchange within a certain time period. Process recordings should also contain your observations of the patient's nonverbal communication. Although different formats may be used for process recording, many people like to record their data in three columns: one for the patient's words, one for the nurse's words, and one for an analysis of the conversation or personal notes.

3. As you study this unit, try to implement the various transcultural communication techniques suggested in the chapters and record how using these techniques helped you to communicate better with your patients.

4. You may also want to concentrate on overcoming one transcultural communication barrier each week. For example, during one week you might decide to focus on *stereotyping*. Recall from Chapter 5 that a cultural stereotype is the unsubstantiated assumption that all people of a certain race or ethnic group are alike. Here are two possible diary entries.

Week of March 18th: Watch Out for Stereotyping

3/18 Today, I was assigned a Jewish patient, and I caught myself thinking that I didn't want to take care of this woman because *all* Jewish patients are very demanding, and her demands were going to interfere with my other patient assignments. I immediately realized that I was making a false assumption. Actually, the patient turned out to be very pleasant and cooperative.

3/21 While I was eating in the hospital cafeteria, a staff nurse remarked that *all* Mexicans eat a lot of fatty foods. He said that refried beans cooked in lard is a daily staple. I said that wasn't true. I told the nurse that I had recently spent some time as a participant-observer in a Mexican community, and I found that *some* Mexicans ate a lot of fatty foods, but many others were watching their fat intake.

5. Remember to keep your diary in a private place. You will not feel as free to write about your transcultural interactions if other people might read your personal thoughts, feelings, and experiences.

CHAPTER 7

Exploring Transcultural Communication As a Participant-Observer

KEY TERMS

- Context
- Ethnography
- Explicit Awareness
- Fieldwork
- Grand-Tour Question
- Key Informant

- Participant Observation
- Rapid Assessment Procedures (RAP)
- Repetitive Social Situation
- Selective Inattention
- Sensory Overload

OBJECTIVES

After completing this chapter, you should be able to:

- Define the components of a repetitive social situation.
- Identify the four phases of participant observation.
- Define the characteristics of each phase of participant observation.
- Discuss the meaning of being an insider and outsider in participant observation.
- Describe the characteristics of a good key informant.

INTRODUCTION

Nurses, like all human beings, are continually engaged in the process of observation. We observe something every second of our conscious lives and process a tremendous amount of information at various levels of awareness. Information remains in our conscious awareness (**explicit awareness**) when we use it to make sense of social situations and to participate in them appropriately.

Through the process of **selective inattention**, information not needed to function appropriately in the immediate environment is sifted out and falls by the cognitive wayside. We just tune it out by not consciously acknowledging it. Selective inattention helps us avoid **sensory overload**, or the inability to process and cope with all of the environmental stimuli we receive (Spradley, 1997a). Selective inattention allows a nurse to give an injection without noting how far away the chair is from the bed, seeing the title of what the patient is reading, noting what color the room is painted, or identifying what is playing on the television. All of those things are present or happening, but they remain out of the nurse's explicit awareness because they are of no consequence to the task at hand.

REPETITIVE SOCIAL SITUATIONS

We learn the verbal and nonverbal behavior expected of us through our observation and participation in **repetitive social situations (RSSs)**, or everyday events that occur over and over again. Repetitive social situations are composed of time, place, person(s), activities, and their interactions (Spradley, 1997a). They recur over time with the same or similar types of individuals and in the same or similar kinds of places (settings). Observation and participation in RSSs helps us learn the cognitive maps (cultural rules for and patterns of behavior expected of us) that allow us to conduct our daily lives, relate to others, and give nursing care with a minimum of misunderstanding, confusion, or conflict.

When some aspect of an RSS changes or is unfamiliar, the persons involved may become confused, uncomfortable, anxious, angry, hostile, or unable to function. More commonly, their selective inattention may prevent them from even realizing a change has occurred; cause them to dismiss it as inconsequential; consider it a misunderstanding, mistake, or ignorance on the part of another; or simply demand that the other person(s) conform to the way things ought to be, do the right thing, or act properly.

Nurse–patient encounters are types of RSSs. Nurses are most comfortable when interacting with patients who share their understanding of what behaviors are expected and act accordingly. When changes occur in some aspect of the usual nurse–patient encounter, nurses and patients may experience discomfort, anxiety, and anger because their expectations of each other have not been met or they have been unable to relate to one another in the usual and heretofore appropriate manner. Our discomfort becomes more pronounced when we must function in a different care setting, such as in patients' homes, neighborhood clinics, or mobile vans. Our selective inattention often causes us to miss important verbal and nonverbal cues in altered or new social situations. These cues can help us identify the rules and patterns of communication behavior in the new setting if we are aware of them.

CONTEXT

All RSSs occur in a **context**. Context consists of the temporal, social, cultural, physical, chemical, biological, and metaphysical environments in which we live and that affect our everyday existence, adaptation, and interaction.

Because of the ever-changing temporal and other aspects of natural settings, contexts are never precisely identical. For example, RSSs occur at different times of the day, week, or year; additional people are present; placement of furniture or equipment varies; the temperature is warmer or colder; or patient needs are different. The ever-changing nature of the context in which RSSs occur requires that all behavior be contextualized; that is, behavior must be viewed and analyzed on the basis of the who, what, when, where, and why of the RSS. Contextualizing behavior helps nurses overcome their selective inattention in RSSs and better understand and adapt to the cultural rules for and patterns of behavior that govern their patient interactions.

• • • COMMUNICATION CONSIDERATIONS • • •

When observing the dynamics of nurse–patient encounters, we need to be like investigative reporters and gather information on the who, what, where, and when of the interaction. *Who* is present? *What* is happening? *Where* is it happening? *When* is it happening? Information from the "Five Ws" will help us understand the "sixth W"—the why (meaning) of the event. *Why* is it happening? Once we get the facts of the story together, we will better understand the cultural rules for and patterns of behavior expected of us when we interact with patients.

Because patient populations are becoming more culturally diverse and the health care environment and modes of care delivery are rapidly changing, we need to develop methods of overcoming selective inattention in order to learn about the cultural beliefs and practices of the populations we serve and the settings in which we practice. It is impossible to learn everything about every cultural group in existence or the variations within each group or RSS. However, we can use modified forms of the anthropological method of **participant observation** (PO) to overcome our selective inattention, contextualize behavior, and gain a relatively rapid understanding of different groups, settings, cultural beliefs and practices, and modes of communication.

PARTICIPANT OBSERVATION

One of the best ways to learn about cultural groups is to observe and interact (participate) with them as they go about their daily lives. We do this naturally when we vacation in other countries, attend ethnic wedding and birthday celebrations, or just sit and talk about life with friends from different ethnic groups. All of these activities help us to better understand and communicate during nurse–patient encounters.

• • • COMMUNICATION CONSIDERATIONS • • •

Learning about multiple aspects of the culture of various ethnic groups is important. Culture is an integrated system of values, beliefs, and practices that stems from a common world view (concept of reality). Culture guides decision making and behavior in all dimensions of life. As you expand your cultural knowledge about a group, you will also enhance your understanding of the beliefs and practices guiding their health behavior.

Everyday Observation and Participant Observation

Nurses, like all human beings, are participants and observers in the realities of their daily existence. However, there are distinct differences between being an ordinary participant in an RSS and being a participant-observer in the anthropological sense (Spradley, 1997b). For example, nurse participant-observers at a well-baby clinic would do the following:

Action	Example
Enter RSS with two objectives: (1) to actively and appropriately engage in the events occurring and (2) to consciously observe the who, what, where, when, and why.	
Seek to overcome their selective inattention and become explicitly aware of information they normally block out.	What are mothers doing while waiting to be seen at well-baby clinics? How does the context affect their behavior?
Use *wide-angle lenses*; that is, pay particular attention to (take mental pictures of) all that is occurring in the RSS and not just focus on what is necessary to accomplish immediate tasks.	Who is present and what is happening at the well-baby clinic while the mothers are waiting to be seen?
Experience how it is to *be both an insider and outsider at the same time* in the RSS.	How do my nurse colleagues and the mothers respond to each others' verbal and nonverbal behavior when they interact? Who initiates the interaction? When and where does it occur? What tone of voice do the nurses and mothers use? Does the nurses' verbal and nonverbal behavior change when there is too little time and too many mothers and infants to see and teach? Do nurses behave differently with mothers from different racial, ethnic, and socioeconomic groups? What happens when I interact with the mothers? Do I act, speak, and feel the same way as my colleagues? Did I behave as a culturally sensitive professional?

Action	Example
Be more *introspective* and use themselves as the *data-gathering instrument* to: (1) determine and understand the cultural rules for and patterns of behavior and (2) gain skill in following those rules by behaving like an insider (native).	Why did I act, say, and feel as I did when I did? Did I behave as the mothers expected me to behave? Did the mothers respond to my behavior as I thought they would?
Interview persons (**key informants**) who are participants in the RSS or others who are experts in patient–staff behavior who can explain what is occurring and why.	Before I leave, I want to talk to some of the nurses and mothers to learn what they did, said, or felt during the RSS that I observed and why. Were they doing, saying, and feeling the same things as I thought on the basis of my observations? What do I need to know to feel more comfortable and to be more effective? How can I get the mothers to ask more questions?
Keep *field notes* (written records) of their objective (what they observe) and subjective observations (what they see, feel, and do) in the RSS. Field notes help to reconstruct and contextualize experiences at a later time.	When I look back over my first month as a nurse participant-observer in the well-baby clinic, do I feel and act differently now than after the first week? What happened to affect my behavior and feelings? Am I more comfortable and better able to interact with and teach the mothers now? Why? When and why did my comfort level change? Are the mothers more willing to listen and respond to me?

In the traditional anthropological method of PO, the anthropologist conducts **fieldwork** (studying and living with a group) for a year or more preparatory to writing an **ethnography**, a description and analysis of a group's culture. Nurses cannot realistically take a year or more to learn the cultural rules for and patterns of behaviors of all of the groups with which they interact. However, aspects of two types of PO can be combined to help us understand how to obtain cultural knowledge about ethnic groups and the settings where we provide care. The traditional four-stage PO process will serve as the framework for the discussion. **Rapid assessment procedures** (RAP), a modified or short-hand version of PO, will be used to demonstrate how nurses can quickly gather information about specific, circumscribed aspects of their patients' cultural beliefs and practices that affect their health (Scrimshaw & Hurtado, 1987).

Phases of Participant Observation

The four phases of the traditional PO process are:

1. complete observer
2. observer as participant
3. participant as observer
4. complete participant

Participant observation is actually a continuum that participant-observers go back and forth on, depending on the nature of the RSS and the depth of their understanding of the cultural rules governing the behavior of those in the RSS. When on the *observation* portion of the continuum, participant-observers are better able to stand aside, see the interactions in the RSS more completely and objectively, and validate information provided by key informants. For example, nurses who observe their colleagues teaching diabetic patients can better evaluate the effectiveness of teaching and learning techniques by using their wide-angle lenses to observe the interactions of their colleagues and patients rather than by doing the teaching themselves. By not actively engaging in the teaching-learning process as insiders, they lessen their selective inattention and personal investment in the success of the teaching endeavor. They can focus more on how aspects of the context affect the teaching-learning process as it unfolds, observe how verbal and nonverbal behaviors of nurses and patients affect their interactions, and talk with participants afterward about their perceptions of the session.

When on the *participation* portion of the continuum, participant-observers can subjectively experience as insiders what those in the RSS are experiencing. They can simultaneously understand the experience from the other persons' points of view and raise additional questions for further PO and confirmation of new cultural knowledge and skills. For instance, nurses who actually go to markets in an ethnic neighborhood can see the types of foods available, evaluate their cost, ask other shoppers and store personnel about what conditions they believe the foods are especially good or bad for, and learn about their preferred preparation. Nurses will be better able to adapt diabetic diets of persons from that ethnic group to the ethnic foods available, their income levels and tastes, and the culturally perceived appropriateness of such foods for diabetics.

When using PO as part of a formal research study, researchers are required to make certain that the persons under study are aware that research is being done, have been apprised of their rights as research participants, and have voluntarily agreed to participate. The ensuing discussion of PO does not encompass all elements of a formal research study. It is merely intended to demonstrate techniques nurses can use to help overcome selective inattention. Nevertheless, it is always a good idea to let people know when and why we are observing them, asking them many questions about their common, everyday activities, and engaging in many of those activities with them.

• • • COMMUNICATION CONSIDERATIONS • • •

If people know you are actively trying to learn more about their culture or their feelings about a situation and you are interested in them as persons, they are more willing to share information with you and to educate you in their cultural beliefs and practices.

Phase One: Complete Observer. The role of a complete observer is like being a spectator who is visible but has no direct interaction with those being observed. The complete observer role is advantageous when we know little, if anything, about a group or the cultural rules for and patterns of behavior governing their interactions. Table 7-1 lists examples of ways you, as a complete observer, can obtain basic background information about multiple dimensions of a group's cultural beliefs and practices. As you do such observations, write notes or memos to yourself (field notes) of questions your observations raise in your mind or any inferences you draw from them or hunches you have about their meaning. At a later time, you can ask key informants about your questions, inferences, and hunches.

TABLE 7-1

Gathering Basic Information about Cultural Groups As a Complete Observer

- Read scholarly texts, articles, reports, or surveys about the cultural group, especially those that deal with health and illness. Most university and public libraries or government agencies have such works available.

- Watch films, television, videos, and stage plays and read fictional novels that deal with the cultural group. (See Appendix II for some ideas.) Foreign language media are an excellent source of such material.

  - Pay particular attention to the context (who, what, where, when, and why) of facial expressions, mannerisms, gestures, and other nonverbal behaviors; tones of voice; gender, spousal, intergenerational, and family roles and relationships; types of health care and resources available; social and welfare issues of importance; cultural meaning and use of food; and formal and informal political processes (what are the politics of what is happening?).

- Read newspapers and literature published by cultural groups to learn about issues of import to them. Such media are found in ethnic neighborhoods at news and book stores; markets and local grocery stores; public transportation stops; restaurants; schools; churches; health care facilities; post offices and other government agencies; gas stations; and auto repair shops.

- Write to national governments of the cultural group's country of origin or call their local consulates or national embassies for information.

- Nurses may also assume a more visible complete observer position similar to being a "fly on the wall" or a loiterer just hanging around. The nurse–observer is removed from the center of action but is able to hear and see what is happening. Table 7-2 gives examples of how a complete observer can learn about the cultural and contextual dimensions of provider–patient interactions in a primary care clinic.

TABLE 7-2

Gathering Information about Provider–Patient Interactions

- Position yourself so that you can observe interactions between health care providers and patients in a primary care facility. Do note the following information and activities.

- To refresh your memory about the RSS later on, draw a map of the physical setting, marking where essential elements are located (e.g., doors, windows, waiting area, reception and work areas, laboratories, examination and diagnostic rooms, refreshment machines area, toilets, audiovisual viewing areas, trash receptacles, and equipment and storage areas).

- Note how the placement of objects (e.g., chairs, desks, and equipment) and the location of rooms, doors, and windows shape, interfere with, or promote effective provider–patient interactions and other types of interpersonal interactions.

- Mark down who the participants are in this RSS and what forms of interactions they have. For example:
  - Who talks and who listens?
  - Was eye contact made and who made it?
  - What was the speed of the conversation and tones of voice used by each participant?
  - What gestures did the participants use?
  - How did the participants carry themselves when walking?
  - What was their posture when sitting?
  - What was their posture when talking to each other?
  - What forms of physical contact took place? How did participants react to such contact?
  - What was the effect on patients when the contact with health care providers was neutral, friendly, or impersonal?
  - Were they standing/sitting close together or far apart?

- Did patients in the waiting area interact with each other?
  - What did they speak about?

- ■ What was their verbal and nonverbal behavior?
- ■ How was their behavior similar and/or different from their behavior when interacting with health care providers?
- ● What was the form and content of health education provided? Who gave it?
- ● Did the health teaching seem clear and understandable?
  - ■ Were questions asked of patients to ascertain their prior understanding of the topic?
  - ■ Were attempts made to confirm that the patient understood the information imparted?

Similar types of observations can be carried out in other types of RSSs in patient care areas and in community settings (Table 7-2). Such observations will generate questions to ask key informants to clarify, confirm, or reject preliminary inferences about contextual factors that affect nurse–patient interactions. They will also provide basic information to explore during other phases of the PO process. This information can be used to further clarify the effects of culture on communication and to ascertain the rules for transcultural communication between ourselves and others in a variety of RSSs.

COMMUNICATION CONSIDERATIONS

Developing wide-angle lens observation skills is especially important when nurses are in a clinical situation in which they know very little, if anything, about the culture of the patient with whom they are about to interact.

When acceptable cultural rules for and patterns of communication behavior are unknown, your best course of action is to follow the patient's lead (Andrews & Boyle, 1997; Villaire, 1994).

Example:
- ● If the patient does not look you in the eyes when speaking, do not look the patient in the eyes. Instead, direct your gaze to wherever the patient is looking (at the floor, to the wall over the right shoulder, or to the top of the desk).

- If the patient speaks slowly and softly, speak the same way.

- If the patient does not firmly grip your hand during a handshake, apply the same type of pressure rather than firmly gripping the patient's hand.

- If the patient defers to a family member when answering your questions, include that family member directly in the patient assessment process.

- If the patient moves closer to you while responding to your question or engaging you in conversation, do not back away out of the patient's comfort zone.

Following patients' leads will convey that you respect them, that you welcome their participation in the assessment process, and that you are willing to learn from them. When it comes to questions about cultural rules for behavior, there is no better way to become competent in the use of culture than for the patient to become the teacher and you the learner.

···· COMMUNICATION CONSIDERATIONS ····

Just observing a series of interactions that are occurring over and over again is one of the best and most unobtrusive ways to gain a beginning knowledge about behavior. You can then raise questions to ask the people involved to learn more about the meaning of what you saw.

Phase Two: Observer as Participant. Observation and interviewing constitute the majority of the participant-observer's time and may be accomplished in two general ways. Nurses continue to observe the RSS, but they also include interviewing of key informants to clarify impressions and inferences they have made from their previous observations. (See Tables 7-1 and 7-2.) A typical sequence of events for this strategy is given in Table 7-3, using the example of patients from a particular cultural group who seldom look directly at health care providers (HCPs) during verbal exchanges. You can use the same strategies in different types of transcultural communication situations.

TABLE 7-3

Data Gathering Using Observation and Interviews

Strategy	Example
Make additional observations in other RSSs to confirm your initial observation.	Members of a cultural group seldom look directly at HCPs during verbal interactions.
Make inferences (best guesses) or hunches regarding the meaning of behavior *and*	"I think it means they are shy with strangers." "It could also be a way to show respect to HCPs."
Jot down questions about the behavior to ask key informants *and*	"Is it due to shyness?" "Is it a way to show respect?" "Is it a form of politeness?" "Does it mean they agree or disagree with HCPs?"
Consult the literature or other sources of data for information about the cultural group.	What have others learned about nonverbal behavior, facial expressions, eye contact, and talking with HCPs?
Interview key informants: First, briefly summarize the inferences/hunch and *then*	Ask the questions about the preliminary inferences/hunches you wrote down. "I have noticed that patients from this cultural group do not look at HCPs when they are speaking. Why is this?"
Based on the explanation given, ask more focused questions to get specific information about aspects of the behavior.	"When is it proper to look directly at someone when talking?" "How does age, gender, or position of authority affect whether they look directly at people when talking?"

(continues)

TABLE 7-3 *(continued)*

Strategy	Example
Summarize the answers of each key informant and confirm them to be sure you have accurately understood them.	"Based on what you said, looking directly at someone means *(summarize each meaning obtained)*."
Make inferences about the behavior you believe members of the cultural group expect of you in various RSSs, and confirm them with your key informants.	"When I do teaching, I should avert my eyes to *(whatever the acceptable cultural behavior is)*." "When I greet patients who are older than me, I should do *(whatever the acceptable cultural behavior is)*."
Test out the newly formed rules for cultural behavior by making repeated observations in a variety of similar RSSs with various types of patients from the same cultural group.	Ask yourself if their behaviors are what you expect based on your newly learned rules for and patterns of cultural behavior.
If the actual behavior is repeatedly inconsistent with expected behavior, note differences and contextualize them. Test them out again by consulting key informants and/or making additional observations.	

It is important to remember that people seldom behave exactly the same, even in seemingly identical or similar RSSs. Before concluding that your newly learned cultural rules for communication are incorrect, contextualize them. Were there things different in the environment that could have accounted for the patient's unexpected behavior?

Example:

- Had the patient waited an exceptionally long period of time to be seen?
- Were others present or not present who normally would or would not have been there?

- Was the interaction in the waiting room rather than in the usual and more private examination room?
- Did the patient have an unpleasant encounter with someone while registering or waiting?
- Did you appear angry when you entered the examination room or when you greeted the patient?

Any one of the above factors or events could influence patients to respond differently (not follow their usual cultural rules for verbal communication).

A second way to be an observer as participant is to begin with interviewing and then follow with observations and participation. This is a good strategy when time is limited, an isolated event is experienced or witnessed that is not likely to recur for a long period of time, or when something happens that arouses your curiosity. It is also an ideal strategy when you are simply interested in learning about some aspect of another cultural group. Examples of PO that start with interviewing follow.

Action	Example
You enter an ethnic restaurant and note that it is decorated in a festive manner and members of the ethnic group seem to be celebrating.	When someone comes to take your order, do the following. • Ask what the festivities are about. • Inquire about which foods you should order so that you join in the celebration like a native. • At some point, ask to speak to a key informant (e.g., the owner, the manager, a staff member, or another patron) so you can obtain a more in-depth explanation of the who, what, where, when, and why of the celebration. • Take the opportunity to learn about the different foods on the menu. For example: ▪ When are they typically eaten? ▪ Are they from any particular region of the country or special subcultural group (socioeconomic class, occupation, or gender)?

Action	Example
	▪ Which foods are considered particularly nutritious and why? ▪ Are they associated with any particular event (e.g., holiday, festival, or family celebration)?

Attend a religious ceremony in an ethnic place of worship. Before going, read about the religion.	Do the following:
	• Note the events occurring, who is participating in them, and how they act.
	• Speak with a key informant (clergy, worshiper, or ritual assistant) to learn about different aspects of the worship service and the religion.
	  ▪ What do the various symbols mean (e.g., dress, items used in the ceremony, coverings on altars or other structures, paintings, statues, texts, singing, and music)?
	  ▪ What special religious services may be done during illness?
	  ▪ Which religious symbols are used to protect or restore the health of a group or individual?
	  ▪ When are members of the ethnic group likely to seek religious help or guidance?
	  ▪ Who can provide such assistance?
	  ▪ What are the special religious holidays and observances of the group?

Go to arts and crafts festivals held by different ethnic groups or to open-air markets in ethnic neighborhoods.	Ask key informants (e.g., booth operators, artisans, festival organizers, or patrons) about some of the following: • What are the history and origin of the festival or market? • What does the art or dance symbolize? • What foods are available? ▪ What do they mean in the context of the festival? (See the restaurant example given earlier.)

- If there is a health component to the festival or market, gather information about the products available, when they are used, and how they are to be prepared.
  - Explore the who, what, where, when, and why of alternative healing modalities that may be on display.

Similar types of interviewing can be done in conjunction with weddings, funerals, births, coming-out ceremonies, sports, recreational and leisure-time events, family gatherings, ethnic pharmacies, and alternative healers or alternative healing establishments.

COMMUNICATION CONSIDERATIONS

Avail yourself of every opportunity to learn about some facet of a group's culture. When learning about cultural characteristics, explore the history of their origin, their meaning, and their relationship to health, illness, and good fortune. It is through endeavors such as these that you can learn the cultural rules for and patterns of behavior as well as the types of cultural resources within an ethnic community that can be utilized in patient care.

Phase Three: Participant As Observer. Because you will already know a great deal about the cultural rules for and patterns of communication behavior, this phase requires less detachment or separation of participant-observers from the events at hand than during phase two. Now, you can refine your knowledge and skills by spending a great deal of time in the participant role. Instead of mainly observing nurse–patient interactions and interviewing key informants in a primary care setting, you can now consciously use the cultural rules for communication behavior that you learned when interacting with and caring for patients.

The participant-as-observer role is a natural progression on the PO continuum. Communication skills and knowledge gained through the observer-as-participant role in phase two becomes the basis for interaction with patients. There are, however, inherent problems in trying to be a participant as observer. Completing the task at hand often assumes primacy. When we are directly giving care, we are often so focused on that task that we forget to be alert to or simply have no time to consciously observe our patients' reactions to us or ours to them. Such involvement in the task at hand severely compromises our ability to step out of our insider's role of caregiver and into the role of outsider so we can objectively critique our behavior as well as that of our patients. Nor do we have the time or freedom to observe events affecting the context in which we are giving care.

Despite the disadvantages inherent in the participant-as-observer role, it is a good way for nurses to test their ability to apply newly learned transcultural communication skills and knowledge. Methods of overcoming problems of doing two jobs at once or serving two masters are listed in Table 7-4.

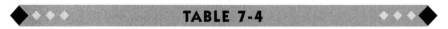

TABLE 7-4

Critiquing the Participant As Observer

- With the permission of the other participants in the RSS, have several of your interactions videotaped. Then critique the videos with key informants.

- With their permission, audiotape your interactions with different types of patients. Critique the tapes with the following questions in mind. You may also want to go over the tapes with a key informant and ask:

  - Am I adapting my teaching and assessment interviews to my patients' characteristics (e.g., level of education, developmental stage, knowledge of conditions, the topic at hand, or concept of privacy)?

  - Did I seek out my patients' knowledge, opinions, beliefs, and/or practices before I began my health teaching or prescribed treatment interventions?

  - Am I picking up verbal and nonverbal cues from my patients that indicate if additional information is needed, the teaching is understood, or the topic is causing distress?

- Have a culturally knowledgeable colleague or someone else observe you as you give care. Discuss their impressions of your ability to apply your transcultural communication skills and knowledge, and your patients' responses.

- As soon as possible after a patient interaction is completed, sit down and write out or tape record all that you can remember about it. Reread your notes/listen to the tape and embellish upon your original account. Then critique the interaction.

Phase Four: Complete Participant. This phase of PO is generally not advocated as a way to begin learning about transcultural communication behavior. Being a complete participant means that nurses would be full-fledged members of the group under study, interact at all levels with all other participants in the RSS, and function in their role as nurses. Full immersion in carrying out work roles and responsibilities increases our selective inattention and constricts our ability to see the RSS through a wide-angle lens. Our tendency is to focus on the immediate tasks needing to be done rather than concentrating on everything else that is occurring in the context. It is just too difficult to be fully immersed in one's daily work while simultaneously being detached enough from it to observe things objectively and to be introspective about our actions, thoughts, and feelings.

The various examples just presented are but a small sample of the variety of ways we can use PO to learn about the rules for and patterns of transcultural communication as well as lifeways of different cultural groups. A variety of other cultural observation exercises can be found in texts by Hunter and Foley (1976), Pedersen (1988), Scrimshaw and Hurtado (1987), and Singelis (1998).

PARTICIPANT-OBSERVATION INTERVIEWING

Interviewing key informants in conjunction with PO is necessary to fully grasp or understand the cultural insider's point of view and the meaning of what is occurring in the RSS and to contextualize it. Interviewing also helps to clarify the basis of differences that may exist between the cultural outsiders' and cultural insiders' perspectives on the RSS. Interviewing can reveal areas in which further cultural knowledge is needed before a cultural outsider can behave in a culturally appropriate manner in an RSS.

When nurses are first learning about a topic, unstructured interviews along the line of friendly conversation are most helpful. The easiest way to learn about a topic is to get people to tell their stories by asking broad-based, open-ended, **grand-tour questions**: "Tell me what you thought was happening when you first began experiencing your symptoms" or "What is it like to have to care for your ill mother at home?" "How did this affect your family?" These would be good types of questions to use in phase two of PO when you start out with interviews rather than observations.

When conducting unstructured, interactive interviews, the main role of nurses is to actively listen and encourage the speaker to continue. This can be done nonverbally via nods of the head, facial expressions, or other gestures. We can also verbally encourage the speaker to go on speaking: "Please, go on." "How interesting. Tell me more." A good way to end such a broad-based or far-ranging interview is to ask, "Is there anything else you can tell me about (whatever the topic is)?" or "What else should I know about (whatever the topic is)?"

Some interviews during the PO process may be more formal; they have a specific purpose and focus and are conducted at a particular time and place, generally of the cultural insider's choice. Such interviews usually occur when interviewers (cultural outsiders) know the questions to ask but cannot predict the answers. Questions should be arranged in a logical order, cover the entire topic of interest, and be semistructured to allow patients to freely describe and explain the situation in their own terms. Examples would be: "Tell me what you do to stay so well" or asking mothers, "Please explain what it means when an infant cries." "What should a mother do when babies cry?" "When is it good for a baby to cry?" For further information on interviewing techniques during PO, see Hunter and Foley, 1976; Morse and Field, 1995; Scrimshaw and Hurtado, 1984; and Spradley, 1997b.

KEY INFORMANTS

The type of key informant may vary with the RSS and phase of PO. Persons who are actually part of the RSS become key informants when participant-observers ask them to explain, clarify, or interpret what they have seen or experienced. At other times, participant-observers may deliberately seek out individuals who can tell them the meaning of what occurred in the RSS even though the key informant was not part of it. For instance, women who have breast-fed can describe how to wean an infant even though they are not presently breast-feeding. They are experts because of their experience.

Certain people make better key informants than others. They are persons who are familiar with the RSS, who are willing to talk about it, and who can discuss what is happening without criticizing it. They accept things as they are and will tell you about a situation without worrying whether it is what ought to be or what they think you want to hear. Additional information about the selection of key informants and their role in PO can be found in the works of Germain (1993) and Spradley (1997b).

REFERENCES

Andrews, M. M., & Boyle, J. S. (1997). Competence in transcultural nursing. *American Journal of Nursing, 97*(8), 16AAA–16DDD.

Germain, C. P. (1993). Ethnography: The method. In P. L. Munhall & C. O. Boyd (Eds.), *Nursing research: A qualitative perspective* (pp. 237–268). New York: National League for Nursing Press.

Hunter, D. E., & Foley, M. B. (1976). *Doing anthropology: A student-centered approach to cultural anthropology.* New York: Harper & Row.

Morse, J. M., & Field, P. A. (1995). *Qualitative research methods for health professionals.* Thousand Oaks, CA: Sage.

Pedersen, P. (1988). *A handbook for developing multicultural awareness.* Alexandria, VA: American Association for Counseling and Development.

Scrimshaw, S. C. M., & Hurtado, E. (1984). Field guide for the study of health seeking behavior at the household level. *Food and Nutrition Bulletin, 6*(2), 27–45.

Scrimshaw, S. C. M., & Hurtado, E. (1987). *Rapid assessment procedures for nutrition and primary health care.* Los Angeles: UCLA Latin American Center Publications.

Singelis, T. M. (Ed.). (1998). *Teaching about culture, ethnicity, and diversity: Exercises and planned activities.* Thousands Oaks, CA: Sage.

Spradley, J. P. (1997a). *The ethnographic interview.* Wadsworth: International Thomson Publishing.

Spradley, J. P. (1997b). *Participant observation.* Wadsworth: International Thomson Publishing.

Villaire, M. (1994). Interview with Toni Tripp-Reimer: Crossing over the boundaries. *Critical Care Nurse, 14*(3), 134–141.

SUGGESTED READINGS

Fetterman, D. M. (1998). *Ethnography: Step by step.* Thousand Oaks, CA: Sage.

Paniagua, F. A. (1994). *Assessing and treating culturally diverse clients.* Thousand Oaks, CA: Sage.

CHAPTER 8

Using Basic Transcultural Communication Techniques

KEY TERMS

- Active Listening
- Empathy
- Exploring
- Feedback
- Focusing
- Mirroring
- Rapport
- Reflecting

- Respect
- Restating
- Self-disclosure
- Sympathy
- Therapeutic Relationship
- Trust
- Validation

OBJECTIVES

After completing this chapter, you should be able to:

- Recognize the importance of transcultural communication in today's health care system.
- Discuss the goals of therapeutic transcultural communication.
- Identify the three phases of a therapeutic relationship, and describe the goals of each phase.
- Select at least five approaches that you can use to establish and increase communication in any transcultural interaction.
- Indicate at least five communication skills that you can use when first meeting a patient from another culture.

INTRODUCTION

Earlier chapters focused primarily on the theory underlying transcultural communication. This chapter will teach you basic transcultural communication techniques that you can use as you work with patients. The importance of clear, sensitive communication during transcultural interactions with patients cannot be overstated. Clear communication is paramount to a harmonious nurse–patient relationship, especially when the nurse and the patient are from very different cultural backgrounds.

This chapter will teach you the basics of communicating successfully with patients from other cultures. You will learn how to:

1. Initiate and build a transcultural, therapeutic nurse–patient relationship.
2. Develop basic transcultural communication skills.
3. Perfect specific transcultural communication techniques.

DEVELOPING A TRANSCULTURAL THERAPEUTIC RELATIONSHIP

Because you will be working closely with patients from different cultures throughout your nursing career, it is very important to learn how to develop a transcultural therapeutic relationship. At first, it may seem difficult to relate in a therapeutic way to people whose cultural beliefs may be very different from your own. Nevertheless, the more you learn about the therapeutic relationship and the more you practice transcultural communication techniques the more skilled you will become. Becoming skillful is an ongoing process.

What Is a Therapeutic Relationship?

A **therapeutic relationship** is an interaction that is directed toward helping a patient heal, both physically and emotionally. Unlike a social relationship, which is based on friendship and mutual interests, a therapeutic relationship is:

- A professional relationship between a nurse, physician, or therapist and a patient.
- Focused on helping the patient solve problems and achieve certain well-defined, mutually agreed-upon, health-related goals.
- A means for more smoothly implementing the five steps of the nursing process: assessing, making a nursing diagnosis, planning, implementing the plan, and evaluating the patient's progress.

- Maintained only as long as the patient requires professional help to meet important health-related goals.

The basic foundation of a therapeutic relationship is *therapeutic communication*. Therapeutic communication is goal oriented. The goals of *transcultural therapeutic communication* are to help patients from different cultures:

1. Explore their life experiences, value and belief systems, and reactions to illness and treatment.

2. Establish realistic, culturally acceptable, health-related goals.

3. Take actions that will benefit their physical and mental health, yet still are in keeping with their personal and cultural values.

Phases of a Therapeutic Relationship

Establishing a therapeutic relationship may take days, weeks, or months. As do all relationships, a therapeutic relationship evolves through different phases. The four major phases of a therapeutic relationship are (Bolander, 1994; Townsend, 2001)

1. The preinteraction phase.

2. The orientation phase.

3. The working phase.

4. The termination phase.

Note: One major difference between a social and a therapeutic relationship is that in the latter a termination phase is inevitable.

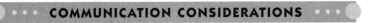

COMMUNICATION CONSIDERATIONS

The successful development of each phase of a therapeutic relationship depends upon the nurse's communication skills.

Preinteraction Phase. During this phase of the relationship, you will need to learn as much as possible about your patient, including reasons for seeking care (see Chapter 11 for detailed information on nursing assessment). To begin your assessment:

- Review the patient's medical record and nursing notes.

- Note the patient's history of previous hospitalizations as well as any procedures that the patient has undergone in the past.

- Note the symptoms that brought the patient to the clinic or hospital.

- Speak with other health care providers who have cared for the patient; inquire about the patient's cultural background and emotional state and the patient's ability to comprehend his or her disorder and its treatment.

In addition to learning about your patient, you also need to think about your own culturally based beliefs and values. Honestly examine yourself for any feelings of bias, prejudice, ambivalence, or hostility that you may harbor toward a patient of a different race or culture. Of course, uncovering these feelings is only the first step in building a transcultural therapeutic relationship. In addition to facing your feelings of prejudice, you must also be able to put these feelings aside when providing care. It is therefore important to increase your awareness of cultural biases and prejudices before the next phases of the nurse–patient relationship.

> **• • • COMMUNICATION CONSIDERATIONS • • •**
>
> Remember that any preconceived negative notions that you may have about a patient can hinder the development of a therapeutic relationship.

Example: A nursing student of Jewish descent had learned as a child that some of her family members had died in the Holocaust. While gathering information about a new patient, the student discovered that this was a non-Jewish person of German descent. The student immediately disliked and distrusted the patient. She also incorrectly presumed that the bias she held against the patient was also held by the patient against her. As a result, the student avoided talking with the patient and failed to gather important assessment data.

The instructor noticed that the student (who was normally very conscientious) had not completed the patient's history and physical examination. The student finally admitted that she felt uncomfortable with the patient because of his German background. The instructor reminded the student that the patient was first and foremost an *individual* like herself. The instructor also pointed out that the student was negatively stereotyping the patient because of his German background. The student agreed to try to put aside her prejudice and preconceived notions. Once the student made an effort to learn about the patient's problems and needs, she began to see him as an individual who was ill and needed her help.

Orientation Phase. During the orientation phase, you need to continue gathering information about your patient's history and current problems. This is also the time to: (1) perform a physical, psychosocial, and cultural assessment; (2) formulate patient outcomes; and (3) plan interventions. Throughout the orientation phase, it is important to show the patient respect and to establish trust and rapport (see pages 147–152). Also, let patients know that confidential material will be shared only with individuals who are directly involved in their care.

Working Phase. As soon as you and the patient have established a therapeutic relationship, the working phase begins. Now you can begin to:

1. Assess the person's concerns, strengths, and weaknesses.

2. Establish a contract with the patient regarding expectations and responsibilities.

3. Decide on mutually agreed-upon goals.

4. Establish a plan of action that satisfies you and the patient.

5. Set limits.

6. Discuss the time frame for your relationship. During this phase, continue to establish rapport and build trust, and, in doing so, encourage the patient to speak openly about feelings, fears, and regrets.

Nursing diagnoses, plans of action, and evaluations may change as a result of your assessment of the patient.

Example: A visiting student from Guatemala was brought into the hospital at the insistence of the American family with whom he was staying. He presented with stomach pains. While the nurse was assessing the patient, the young man insisted that he wanted to go home without seeing the physician. The nurse diagnosed the patient as noncompliant.

However, as the nurse asked more questions about health care in Guatemala, she learned that only acute illnesses are considered worthy of treatment. This patient did not view his pain as acute and in need of medical attention. Because the patient refused treatment owing to his cultural background, the nurse stopped insisting that he wait for a physician. Instead, she had the young man sign a release, instructed him to closely monitor his pain, and advised him to return to the hospital immediately should the pain worsen.

Termination Phase. A therapeutic relationship may be terminated for a variety of reasons: The patient may be discharged; the nurse or nursing student may change services, or the patient's health goals may be met. Regardless of the reason for termination, it should not come as a surprise to the patient. Remember that one of the tasks of the orientation phase is to set a time frame for the relationship and to make certain that the patient understands that the relationship will eventually end. So the termination process needs to be initiated in the orientation phase.

During the termination phase, your major tasks are to:

- Outline the patient's strengths and discuss the progress the person has made while in your care.
- Review areas in need of improvement.
- Discuss the patient's new goals and develop a plan of self-care for the patient after discharge.
- Discuss any feelings (positive or negative) that the patient might have regarding the termination of your relationship.

DEVELOPING TRANSCULTURAL COMMUNICATION SKILLS

Since the 1980s, thousands of immigrants requiring medical and nursing services have arrived in the United States. To work with these culturally diverse groups of patients, nurses need strong transcultural communication skills. Nurses must know how to communicate clearly with people who speak different languages and whose cultural backgrounds, values, lifestyles, traditions, and expectations differ (however subtly) from their own.

Although you cannot be knowledgeable about every cultural group, it is important to identify the cultural variations that could affect your communication with patients. For example, you should recognize that people from different cultures:

- Differ in their cultural heritage and thus in their perceptions of illness and treatment.
- Have unique ways of viewing and interacting with health care providers; for example, refugees who have been subjected to imprisonment or torture may view doctors and nurses as dangerous authority figures.
- Regard some forms of verbal and nonverbal communication as appropriate and other forms as not appropriate. Recall from Chapter 4 that some Asians and Native Americans may regard prolonged eye contact as rude.

• • • • COMMUNICATION CONSIDERATIONS • • • •

The key to successful transcultural communication is to recognize the uniqueness of every culture, every relationship, and every individual—including yourself.

Also, people from different cultures who are ill may have different ways of communicating their fears and needs. Patients may become anxious, resistant, resentful, distrustful, or offended when they feel that a nurse does not respect their customs, needs, and feelings. A nurse can become frustrated and even angry when patients disregard instructions because of a failure to understand or accept the nurse's verbal and nonverbal communications.

Example: A patient who had recently immigrated from Thailand was scheduled for a CT scan. While explaining the procedure to the patient, the nurse often touched the patient's head to illustrate that the procedure might cause a severe headache. Suddenly, during this demonstration, the patient became withdrawn and anxious. Appearing to be deeply offended, the patient refused to listen further to the nurse, and he also refused the procedure.

The nurse felt angry, frustrated, and confused. Unfortunately, the nurse did not realize that in many Asian cultures, the head is a sacred part of the body, and it is considered the carrier of the soul. Thus, the nurse failed to understand that her actions had insulted the patient and devalued his cultural beliefs. Had the nurse been culturally competent, she would have demonstrated her point with an illustration of a person's head or pointed to her own head. This simple technique would have helped to establish transcultural communication, and the patient would have undergone the procedure.

Establishing Transcultural Communication

Before you can initiate and build a therapeutic relationship, assess patients, or plan and provide their care, you must first establish communication. In other words, your patients must be willing to talk with you, listen to your questions, and give you honest answers. They must trust you enough to tell you about their health history, symptoms, problems, and stresses. They must be willing to listen to your suggestions and follow your instructions. Communicating with patients from different cultures requires sensitivity, knowledge, and skills that can be acquired with study, practice, and experience.

Remember that talking with relative strangers about deeply personal issues is never easy, and it can be particularly difficult for patients who are from different cultural backgrounds than the nurse or physician. To encourage patients to talk to you about themselves, you must first

1. Convey empathy.
2. Show respect.
3. Build trust.
4. Establish rapport.
5. Listen actively.
6. Provide appropriate feedback.
7. Demonstrate genuine interest.

Conveying Empathy. **Empathy** involves actively sharing another person's feelings. Empathy can be described as taking on the role of another and experiencing what that person is experiencing. It is not the same as **sympathy**, an emotion that involves feeling sorry for someone. Empathy is allowing yourself to enter into another person's emotional experience while, at the same time, maintaining objectivity and carrying out your role as the nurse.

> **• • • COMMUNICATION CONSIDERATIONS • • •**
>
> It is important for nurses to be empathetic while still maintaining a professional relationship with their patients.

Example: An empathetic nurse is able to share the painful emotions of a patient who has just received a breast cancer diagnosis while *simultaneously* helping the person make arrangements for surgery. Unfortunately, because of their own anxieties, some nurses are unable to share in the feelings of others and, instead, distance themselves from their patients' painful emotions. For example, an anxious nurse might efficiently schedule a patient's breast surgery but avoid talking with the patient about the disturbing implications of a cancer diagnosis. This distancing on the part of the nurse can greatly weaken the bonds of a therapeutic relationship.

Showing Respect. Patients want and need to be treated with respect. **Respect** is more than simply accepting another person; respect is valuing another person and viewing that individual as special. To help patients feel that you respect them, begin by interacting with patients in a formal manner. Members from many Asian and Hispanic cultures respond particularly well to a formal approach to history taking, assessment, and care. It is also important to show respect for the patient's personal space and status. Enabling patients to observe their religious practices and holidays also demonstrates respect.

Older patients, regardless of culture, deserve to be treated respectfully. For instance, although it is a common practice, it is not respectful to address older men or women by their first name or by a nickname unless they give you permission to do so. Older people from cultures that hold elders in high esteem may particularly resent being addressed by their first name.

COMMUNICATION CONSIDERATIONS

When you listen to your patients and respect their cultural values and beliefs, you are more likely to gain their trust and cooperation. As a result, patients will be more willing to talk with you about symptoms and problems and also more motivated to follow your suggestions and instructions.

Building Trust. **Trust** involves having confidence or faith in another person. Trust is a vital component of the nurse–patient therapeutic relationship. Patients who trust you will feel confident that you will watch after their best interests and that you will respect their right to privacy and confidentiality. Patients will also feel comfortable discussing their symptoms with you and even disclosing intimate details of their lives.

However, culture can influence how many personal details a patient is willing to share with care providers. For example, Asians typically value a subtle approach to the discussion of problems, and they tend to restrain the expression of strong feelings. Thus, Asian patients may find it difficult to speak openly with their nurses about any mental health problems and may tend to express emotional distress in terms of physical complaints. Refugees may view you as an authority figure and thus as a person who cannot be trusted.

COMMUNICATION CONSIDERATIONS

To establish trust with patients, promise no more than you can deliver, keep appointments, and carefully explain procedures and policies—with the help of an interpreter if necessary.

Establishing Rapport. Establishing rapport results in gaining your patient's trust and acceptance. **Rapport** is manifested through warmth and friendliness and the feeling that the two people are comfortable with each other. To establish rapport with a patient, you might begin by discussing non-health-related topics. For example, you might ask a foreign patient where he is from, how long he has lived in the United States, and how he likes living here. If the patient appears comfortable with these initial questions, you can then discuss the person's present symptoms and medical history.

Listening Actively. **Active listening** consists of giving verbal and non-verbal clues that communicate that you are interested in the patient. When you actively listen to your patient, you build trust and show respect. The acronym SOLER is sometimes used to describe the techniques that promote active listening.

S. *Sit* facing the patient. This position sends the message that you want to listen to the patient, and it tells the person that you are interested in what is being said.

O. Maintain an *open posture*. Sit with your hands in your lap and your legs uncrossed in a relaxed posture that is nonauthoritative and nonthreatening. This posture signifies openness, and it will encourage your patient to speak freely. Sitting or standing with your hands on your hips or your arms crossed in front of you is a more authoritative stance that may inhibit the patient or evoke a defensive response.

L. *Lean* toward the patient throughout the conversation. This behavior conveys genuine concern and interest. By leaning toward the patient, you are showing that you are attentive and that you sincerely want to understand what the patient is trying to tell you.

E. Establish and maintain *eye contact*. Eye contact conveys interest, whereas avoiding eye contact can convey a lack of interest, disrespect, or boredom. Eye contact in the absence of friendliness may give the impression of disapproval. Also, remember that different cultures react to eye contact differently, so you may need to change your communication style accordingly (see Chapter 4).

R. *Relax.* Sit comfortably in your chair and smile in a friendly manner. Communicating a relaxed attitude will help establish a comfortable nonthreatening environment in which the patient will feel free to speak with you about problems and concerns.

Providing Feedback. Providing a patient with **feedback** (information) concerning a modifiable behavior (e.g., disregarding instructions) can help the person change that behavior. Townsend (2001) lists some important points to remember about feedback.

1. Feedback should be used to *describe a behavior* but not to evaluate (or criticize) the patient. In other words, feedback needs to focus on the *behavior* and not on the person. Evaluating or criticizing can put a person on the defensive, a result that defeats the purpose of feedback.

   Example:
   Evaluation of the person: "Why aren't you cooperating with us? You know that you're supposed to go to physical therapy every day!"
   Description of a behavior: "My nursing assistant mentioned that you didn't want to go to physical therapy. Can you tell me why you didn't feel like going?"

2. Feedback should be *specific* rather than general. Making broad, general statements about the patient's behavior is not helpful. Instead, focus on the *details* of a behavior that the patient can modify.

   Example:
   Broad statement: "According to your wife, you are not following your low-calorie diet."
   More detailed feedback: "According to your wife, you are still eating a lot of refried beans instead of the black beans we recommended, which are much lower in calories."

3. Feedback should focus on behaviors or situations that the patient can realistically modify.

   Example:
   Cannot be modified: "You are at risk of high blood pressure because you are a black man."
   Can be modified: "You are at risk of high blood pressure because you are a black man and you are 30 pounds overweight."

4. Feedback should *provide information* rather than advice. Informative feedback encourages patients to sort out information and come to a decision on their own.

   Example:
   Providing advice: "If you really want to lose weight, you should join Weight Watchers."

Providing information: "If you want to lose weight, I can give you a list of the many excellent weight-loss programs that are available. If you call the programs that you are interested in, they will give you all of the details."

5. Provide feedback *as soon as possible* after a specific behavior.

   Example:

   Delayed feedback: "I noticed last week that you did not bring your daughter into the clinic for her reevaluation."

   Timely feedback: "I'm calling you because I didn't see your daughter at the clinic this morning. We would like to see her this afternoon or first thing tomorrow. Can you bring your daughter in?"

Demonstrating Genuine Interest. You can demonstrate genuine interest through *verbal and nonverbal expressions.* Words of concern to the patient can communicate that you are interested in the total well-being of the patient. A caring attitude as expressed in gentle touch and an open posture will communicate to the patient that you are sincere in providing care. It is important to remember that certain behaviors of the nurse may not be acceptable or appropriate for some cultural groups. For example, some patients may perceive an open posture as threatening or as invasive of their personal space and privacy, whereas a nurse who addresses a patient with proper titles, such as "Dr." or "Mrs.," communicates respect and honor to the person.

Using Specific Transcultural Communication Techniques

As you begin your relationship with a patient from another culture, plan to use the following basic transcultural communication techniques (Bolander, 1994; Townsend, 2001):

1. When first meeting a new patient, *approach slowly* and wait for the patient to acknowledge you. Rushing in may exacerbate the fear of the unknown and the unexpected that many patients from other cultures associate with hospitals and health care personnel.

2. *Greet the patient respectfully.* Refer to the patient by title (Dr., Mr., Mrs.) and last name rather than by first name. Make sure that you are pronouncing the patient's name correctly. Also, help the patient pronounce your name if you notice difficulty in doing so.

3. Provide the patient with a *quiet setting* where you will not be disturbed. If the patient is confined to bed, draw the curtains completely around the bed to provide privacy. Patients from some cultures may want their family present.

4. Sit a comfortable distance away and *lean slightly* toward the patient. Do not interrupt the patient. Avoid changing the subject. Nod occasionally; ask pertinent questions to draw the patient out; and—with gestures and facial expressions—indicate that you accept the patient's feelings of anxiety, fear, or anger.

5. If your patient seems uneasy, pull up a chair and position yourself parallel to and lower than the patient. This position helps the patient feel more in control. You may also appear to be more supportive.

6. Allow *sufficient time* for your meeting. Try not to appear rushed or anxious to leave. Avoid fidgeting or looking at the clock. A hurried attitude on your part could offend Hispanic or Asian patients, who value politeness, or Native American patients, who value an unhurried approach to communication. For example, when assessing a Native American patient, do not initially ask questions in a rapid manner. Try a gentler, slower approach. First, identify yourself and then state your name, position, and how long you have worked in the agency or facility. Next, tell the patient what you hope to do and *then* ask questions. Shake hands at the end, not at the beginning of your meeting.

7. *Explain* to patients (especially those who are nervous or fearful) that they can and need to speak freely to you about their symptoms and fears. Emphasize that the information they impart will be shared only with other health care professionals for purposes of diagnosis and treatment.

8. *Listen* to what your patients are trying to tell you about their symptoms. Listen with particular care to the words a patient uses to describe a symptom. Then use those same terms, rather than medical jargon, when discussing symptoms with that patient.

9. Offer the patient opportunities to *ask questions*. For example, as you talk with the patient, periodically pause to inquire: "Would you like to add something?" or "Do you have any further suggestions?" or "How do you feel about this problem?" This approach should help to increase the exchange of information between you and your patient.

However, culture once again influences whether a patient will be quiet during the assessment process or will assertively ask questions. For example, many mainstream white American patients may want to know as much as possible about their condition.

Conversely, out of respect, some Asian patients may hesitate to question a nurse or physician about their diagnosis. However, these Asian patients may still want to know more about their illness. Physicians and nurses need to provide patients with essential information about their diagnosis, even though some patients may not ask direct questions.

10. Try **self-disclosure** to help establish rapport. For example, if the patient is suffering from insomnia, you might mention that sometimes you too are unable to sleep and you understand how distressing insomnia can be.

COMMUNICATION CONSIDERATIONS

Remember that you should use self-disclosure only to help your patient feel more comfortable about providing you with personal information. Once you have established rapport and the patient seems comfortable, you should stop talking about yourself and return the focus of your discussion to your patient.

11. Use **mirroring** as another technique to make communication flow more easily. If the patient is a Native American who speaks slowly and softly, incorporate that aspect of the patient's communication style into your own style. Project calmness in your voice and manner even though you may normally speak rapidly. You might also mirror the person's use of eye contact, increasing or decreasing eye contact as appropriate for that culture.

12. **Focusing** on a single idea or experience mentioned by the patient and then **exploring** it further are two important communication techniques. Delving into experiences, emotions, or ideas in depth helps patients who are hesitant to explore certain subjects on their own. Although the patient may initially find it difficult to talk about a topic, your interest should help the person discuss the matter and disclose feelings more openly.

Example:

Nurse (focusing): Yesterday you mentioned that you were a political prisoner in Tibet before coming to this country. It would be helpful to learn more about your experiences.

Patient: Why should I talk to you about what they did to me and my family? No one believes the torture I've been through.

Nurse (exploring): I realize that you have suffered a great deal. I'm very interested in learning more about you and your family and about how you survived and came to this country. Perhaps we could start by talking about just one incident from your past.

13. **Restating**, or *paraphrasing*, what the patient has said gives the person an opportunity to rethink a statement or idea and then clarify or change the statement. For example, the patient who survived torture might say, "I have terrible nightmares every night. Because of these dreams, I can never forget what they did to me." The nurse could respond by restating, or paraphrasing, the patient's words: "Even though you survived, your dreams make you feel as if you're still a victim."

14. *Seeking* **validation** (confirmation) from a patient ensures that you and your patient are talking about the same thing.
    Example:
    Young black patient: My doctor is really bad!
    White nurse: Do you mean that your doctor is doing a poor job?
    Young black patient: No! My doctor's great! Black people sometimes say *bad* when they really mean *good. Being bad* is a compliment.

15. **Reflecting** questions or statements back to your patients helps to validate their concerns and fosters confidence. No one wants to be misunderstood, and reflecting shows that you understand and recognize the patient's concerns.
    Example:
    Patient: Should I still use this copper bracelet for my arthritis pain?
    Nurse (reflecting back the question): Do you still want to use the copper bracelet? (At this point, the nurse should pause and give the patient time to think and respond.)

16. Allow *silence* as a communication technique when appropriate (see Chapter 4). Silence gives your patient time to reflect and speak. However, patients sometimes use silence to avoid disclosing information about themselves or as a way to control others. Patients who belong to certain religious groups are sometimes silent because they believe that they are listening to and communicating with God (Davidhizar & Giger, 1994).

Davidhizar and Giger suggest these techniques for responding to a patient's silence:

- Avoid interrupting the silence because silence makes you uncomfortable.

- Analyze the meaning of the silence. In the meantime, assess the patient's nonverbal communication, including the person's posture, amount of eye contact, facial expressions, and signs of anxiety.

- Let the patient know that you accept the silence. If the patient looks thoughtful, you might say: "You seem very quiet. I would like to share your thoughts." If the patient looks annoyed or angry, try this approach: "You seem upset. Perhaps we can talk about what is troubling you."

- Provide support if the patient acts anxious or fearful. "I can tell that you don't feel like talking right now. That's all right. I'll just sit here with you for a few minutes." This statement may help the patient to relax.

- Be silent yourself, and let the patient initiate conversation. Sitting quietly with a patient may encourage the person to break the silence and communicate verbally with you.

Although there are many reasons for a patient's silence, members of some groups (especially Native Americans, Southeast Asians, and individuals from an impoverished background) may not speak because they feel discriminated against or misunderstood. Other patients may feel obligated to keep personal and family concerns private. In this case, reassure the patient that you will keep information confidential. Tell your patient that you know it is difficult to disclose personal information. To establish rapport and reduce the patient's feelings of vulnerability, you might want to disclose some of your own experiences and feelings.

Despite your best efforts, some patients may continue to be guarded and silent. In these cases, you may just have to wait for the person to decide that you are worthy of trust. You may need to defer your questions to a later time.

17. Pay attention to the patient's *nonverbal communication* and its cultural significance. If you are from a different culture than your patient, it may be difficult for you to interpret the meaning of nonverbal communication cues, including:

- Quality and tone of voice

- Posture
- Gestures
- Facial expressions
- Use of personal space
- Use of touch
- Frequency of eye contact
- Use of communication that is vocal but still nonverbal such as sighing, crying, laughing, moaning, and coughing

Evaluate the patient's verbal communication and nonverbal signals. When verbal and nonverbal signals do not agree (e.g., the patient says he is not nervous but is clearly trembling), ask additional questions to clarify the person's verbal response.

Take care that your normal nonverbal communication does not unintentionally frighten or offend patients from other cultures. As mentioned, mirroring the communication style of your patients is one technique for building trust and reducing the patient's anxiety.

COMMUNICATION CONSIDERATIONS

Remember that patients from other cultures may be particularly sensitive to your use of touch and eye contact.

18. *Touch* patients only when you know touching is acceptable. As mentioned earlier, the issue of physical contact is indeed touchy. Recall that cultures differ radically as to what kinds of touch are permitted and when. In general, it is more acceptable to touch a child in a comforting manner than an adult. To minimize potential problems, follow these specific guidelines:
    - Many Hispanic patients are accustomed to supportive touch or a gentle embrace. Make a point of shaking hands with Hispanic patients and their families and of standing or sitting close to the patient. It is usually all right to touch a Hispanic patient when paying a compliment, because touch is viewed as a gesture of sincerity. When talking to a Hispanic child, praise and smile while you gently touch the head or hand of the child.
    - Avoid touching a Vietnamese, Cambodian, Hmong, or Thai child on the head during an initial conversation or assessment, because the head has traditionally been considered the site of the soul in these cultures.

- When touching adolescents, tapping the shoulder or touching the hand is considered appropriate, especially for Filipino, Chinese, Japanese, Southeast Asian, and Hispanic youths. These adolescents are inclined to exchange hugs amongst themselves, but males may consider obvious signs of emotion as threats to their masculinity.
- Because the Southeast Asian patient may fear bodily intrusion, minimize touching and probing. Carefully explain assessment and treatment techniques before intruding on the patient.

19. Remember that the accepted amount of *eye contact* differs among cultures. For example, a lack of eye contact that may indicate emotional problems in a typical American child, may be culturally normal for a child from an Asian household. To help you correctly interpret nonverbal clues, ask the interpreter if the child's behavior is acceptable within the culture or if the behavior is unique to the child.

Also, recall from Chapter 4 that white Americans generally view eye contact as symbolic of self-confidence, honesty, integrity, and attentiveness, whereas a lack of eye contact shows disinterest, rudeness, arrogance, and dishonesty. Most Americans and Hispanics are comfortable with eye contact, whereas Asians and Native Americans tend to see eye contact as invasive and a threat to their privacy.

REFERENCES

Bolander, V. B. (1994). *Sorenson & Luckmann's basic nursing: A psychophysiologic approach.* Philadelphia: Saunders.

Davidhizar, R., & Giger, J. N. (1994). When your patient is silent. *Journal of Advanced Nursing, 20*(4), 703–706.

Townsend, M. C. (2001). *Psychiatric mental health nursing: Concepts of care* (5th ed.). Philadelphia: Davis.

SUGGESTED READINGS

Axtell, R. E. (1993). *Do's and taboos around the world* (3rd ed.). New York: Wiley.

Chester, B., & Holtan, N. (1992). Working with refugee survivors of torture. (Cross-cultural medicine—A decade later). *Western Journal of Medicine, 157* [Special issue], 301–304.

Cravener, P. (1992). Establishing therapeutic alliance across cultural barriers. *Journal of Psychosocial Nursing, 30*(12), 10–14.

Fairlie, A. (1992). Nurse–patient communication barriers. *Senior Nurse, 12*(3), 40–43.

Giger, J. N., & Davidhizar, R. E. (2003). *Transcultural nursing: Assessment and intervention* (4th ed.). St. Louis: Mosby.

Kirkham, S. R. (1998). Nurses' descriptions of caring for culturally diverse clients. *Clinical Nursing Research, 7*(2), 125–146.

Meadows, J. L. (1991). Multicultural communication. Sections of this paper were presented at a Maternal and Child Health Conference on *The Meaning of Culture in Health Care* at the University of Illinois at Chicago College of Associated Health Professions.

Purnell, L. D., & Paulanka, B .J. (2003). *Transcultural health care: A culturally competent approach* (2nd ed.). Philadelphia: Davis.

Rankin, S. B., & Kappy, M. S. (1993). Developing therapeutic relationships in multicultural settings. *Academic Medicine, 68*(11), 826–827.

Setness, P. A. (1998). Culturally competent healthcare. *Postgraduate Medicine, 103*(2), 13–16.

Spector, R. E. (2004). *Cultural diversity in health and illness* (6th ed.). Upper Saddle River, NJ: Prentice Hall.

CHAPTER 9

Overcoming Transcultural Communication Barriers

KEY TERMS

- Bias
- Dual Ethnocentrism
- Expectation
- Knowledge Deficit
- Language Barrier
- Medical Terminology

- Multiple Realities
- Participant Observation
- Perception
- Perspective
- Stereotype
- Terminology

OBJECTIVES

After completing this chapter, you should be able to:

- Acquire information about the beliefs and values of the specific cultural groups represented in your patient population.
- Challenge any cultural biases or ethnocentric attitudes that may interfere with your transcultural communication.
- Explain medical terminology to patients from other cultures in terms that they can understand.
- Identify and overcome differences in how you and your patient perceive illness and health care.
- Identify and overcome differences between what you expect and what the patient expects of the Western medical health care system.

INTRODUCTION

Communicating with patients from different cultures may be complicated by (1) the nurse's lack of knowledge; (2) bias, ethnocentrism, prejudice, and stereotyping; (3) language differences; (4) differences in terminology; and (5) differences in perceptions and expectations (see Chapter 5). The sections that follow contain guidelines for overcoming each of these barriers.

OVERCOMING A KNOWLEDGE DEFICIT

Nurses often diagnose their patients as suffering from a **knowledge deficit**. However, nurses themselves may lack important information and knowledge, particularly concerning the cultural groups with whom they work. The nurse who is not knowledgeable about a patient's cultural values, health beliefs, and patterns of seeking help will not be able to provide the culturally sensitive care that all patients deserve.

Fortunately, there are several ways for nurses to learn more about specific cultures. First of all, you can attend classes and seminars that provide valuable information about transcultural nursing. Also, many textbooks are available that describe the history, beliefs, and practices of the major American cultural groups. For example, Chapter 2 in this book discusses the traditional beliefs and values of the mainstream white American, Asian, Hispanic, black, and Native American cultures. However, although textbooks present the facts, they often do not provide the flavor and essence of a culture. The cultural information provided by textbooks must be used only as a framework to guide the practitioner in understanding the beliefs and practices of the patient. This information must be validated during the nurse–patient cultural encounter in the health care setting.

To delve deeper into the heart of a culture, read novels, short stories, biographies, autobiographies, essays, and poems written by members of the cultural group. Documentaries, films, and television programs that portray different cultures; foreign films; and films that are written, produced, and directed by members of these groups can also broaden your appreciation of America's diverse cultures. (See Appendix II for examples.) In addition, many cultural or ethnic groups, such as blacks, Hispanics, and Asians, have their own newspapers, magazines, and radio and television stations that present pertinent issues as well as entertainment. The Internet is another valuable tool for learning more about different cultural groups. (See Chapter 7 for more details on these methods for gathering information.)

In addition to reading, listening to, and viewing information about different cultures, you will also need to involve yourself in a chosen culture as a participant-observer. Recall from Chapter 7 that **participant observation**

(PO) is a modified form of an anthropological method for gaining a relatively rapid understanding of different groups, settings, cultural beliefs and practices, and modes of communication. Chapter 7 provides detailed instructions on how to gather information as (1) a complete observer, (2) a participant as observer, (3) an observer as participant, and (4) a complete participant.

CONTROLLING BIAS, ETHNOCENTRISM, PREJUDICE, AND STEREOTYPING

Bias, ethnocentrism, prejudice, and stereotyping are barriers to transcultural communication because each acts to distort our perception of other cultures (Urden, Stacy & Lough, 2001). In Chapter 5, we defined **bias** as the tendency to view one's own cultural values as better than the cultural values of other people. According to Agar (1996), it is impossible for nurses to completely overcome their personal biases when caring for patients from different cultures. What nurses can do, however, is to bring their biases to consciousness and then try to control those biases when working with patients (Charonko, 1992).

> **Example:** Many nurses educated in the United States are heavily biased toward Western medicine. When caring for a patient from a different culture, American nurses need to acknowledge the *patient's* traditional health care beliefs and permit the patient to follow those beliefs, provided they do not interfere with the patient's medication and treatment program. If the patient's health practices conflict with Western medical practices, the nurse should explain the problem to the patient and then make adjustments that will be *mutually acceptable* to the patient and the nurse.

Nurses must also recognize that "**multiple realities** operate simultaneously in any health care situation" (DeSantis, 1994). In Chapter 5, we introduced the concept of **dual ethnocentrism**, which involves the nurse's assessing and evaluating the patient's cultural beliefs at the same time that the patient is evaluating the nurse's beliefs. According to DeSantis, these nurse–patient encounters involve the interaction of three separate cultures or realities:

1. The **nurse's** professional knowledge, based on an education in Western medicine, as well as personal beliefs and practices.
2. The **patient's** view of Western medicine, based on cultural background and beliefs.
3. The **setting** in which the patient and the nurse are interacting: for example, the hospital, clinic, community, or home and family

setting. Institutions such as these have their own rules and expectations about the responsibilities and standards of care that affect the nurse–patient relationship.

The nurse who understands these multiple realities should be able to view patients from diverse cultures in a clearer light. For instance, patients whom nurses have labeled as *noncompliant* may simply be adhering to their own cultural beliefs rather than to hospital policy and the nurse's biomedical beliefs.

••• COMMUNICATION CONSIDERATIONS •••

Acknowledging that patients have the right to their own health care beliefs is a major step toward overcoming personal and professional biases and ethnocentrism.

Overcoming the tendency to **stereotype** people from different cultures is also very important. Catch yourself before you make statements such as "*All* blacks do this . . . ," "Mexicans *always* do that . . . ," and "Native Americans *never* understand this . . ." In addition, gently correct other nurses when they make stereotypical statements about patients with different racial or ethnic backgrounds.

Example: Kathy Ballard (the evening charge nurse) is giving her report to Ken Nickols (the night nurse).

Kathy: Ken, we just admitted Maria Sanchez again. She's a 62-year-old woman with congestive heart failure. She understands a little English, but she only speaks Spanish.

Ken: So we'll need to find an interpreter to help with her assessment.

Kathy: Definitely. (Sighing) I don't know about you, but I get so tired of people who immigrate to this country and then they don't learn the language—and then we have to find interpreters! It seems like the Mexicans, in particular, never bother to learn English.

Ken: Well, I haven't worked in this hospital as long as you have, Kathy, but my experience has been different. I've met many Mexican patients who speak very good English.

Kathy: Why don't they all learn to speak English?

Ken: Kathy, listen to yourself! Many Mexicans work two jobs in order to support their families here and help out their families in

Mexico. They don't have the time or the money or the energy for English lessons. They have more urgent priorities than learning English.

Kathy: OK, OK, you've made your point. I admit that many Mexicans do speak English, and I guess those that don't have their reasons. I'll call for an interpreter. Why don't you go in and meet Ms. Sanchez. She's probably getting anxious.

OVERCOMING LANGUAGE BARRIERS

Of all the hurdles that nurses and their patients must clear in order to communicate, **language barriers** are possibly the most difficult. Language barriers can create many frustrating problems.

- Language barriers can make it difficult or impossible to obtain a patient's history and assess the patient's symptoms.

- Language barriers can interfere with explaining hospital policies and medical procedures.

- Language barriers can severely impede the vital processes of teaching and counseling the patient and family.

- Language barriers can create misunderstandings and resentments between nurses and patients.

It is so important to learn how to overcome language barriers, that this book devotes an entire chapter to the subject. Chapter 10 will give you clear guidelines for communicating with patients who have limited English proficiency. That chapter also discusses the patient's legal right to have an interpreter as well as the complex role of the medical interpreter.

OVERCOMING TERMINOLOGY DIFFERENCES

In addition to language barriers, communication problems also arise when patients and nurses use different terminology. Most patients—regardless of cultural background—find it difficult to discuss their health problems in the precise clinical terms used by nurses and other health care professionals. First of all, patients tend to focus comments on their discomfort ("It hurts to move my shoulder"), whereas nurses focus on the resulting functional limitations such as "impaired physical mobility related to arthritis."

Furthermore, patients often describe their ailments in highly personalized and often emotional terms such as *the dreaded pest, my high blood pressure, my heart attack,* or *my sugar diabetes.* These terms contrast to the biomedical terms *influenza, hypertension, acute myocardial infarction,* and *diabetes mellitus.*

Stokes (1977) compiled the following list of medical terms that are used by nurses and compared them with equivalent terms used by some black patients (Cherry & Geiger, 1995).

Medical Term	Equivalent Black Term
Pain	Miseries
Syphilis	Bad blood, pox
Anemia	Low blood, tired blood
Vomiting	Throwing up
Constipation	Locked bowels
Diarrhea	Running off, grip
Menstruation	Red flag, the curse
Urinate, urine	Pass water, tinkle; peepee

• • • • COMMUNICATION CONSIDERATIONS • • • •

Listen to the terms that your patient uses and use those terms when performing your assessment. Avoid using abbreviations such as TPR and MI without explaining to the patient what they mean.

Gibbs and associates (1987) studied patients' ability to understand **medical terminology**. Their results indicated that patients do not make the cultural jump from lay to medical terms easily. Nearly 50% of patients randomly selected in an urban primary care center defined *hypertension* as meaning nervousness or being upset. One-quarter of the sampled patients understood *orally* to mean when to take a medication (for example, on the hour) rather than as meaning to take a medication by mouth.

• • • • COMMUNICATION CONSIDERATIONS • • • •

Patients who have difficulty with English may be particularly confused by medical terms.

Unfortunately, busy health care professionals sometimes fail to explain medical terms to patients. Indeed, it is not unusual for physicians and nurses to talk "over the heads" of patients as they perform their assessment. This practice can produce feelings of anxiety, fear, and anger—especially in patients who do not speak English fluently. Such negative feelings can result in patients' noncompliance with important treatment recommendations.

Example: Marie Kowalsky, a young mother and a Polish immigrant who had lived in the United States for four years, brought her 5-year-old daughter to a pediatric clinic. Ms. Kowalsky knew some English, but it was difficult for her to explain her daughter's symptoms to the physician and nurse who were examining the child. During the examination, Ms. Kowalsky unsuccessfully tried to communicate her experience of her child's illness, while the health professionals were more concerned with communicating their observations—primarily to each other.

Ms. Kowalsky (referring to her daughter): Iwona feels bad. She tells me her head hurts. She cry very hard. She cry all the time. I think her ears hurt.

Physician: Let's have a look at her ears. (He begins to examine the child's ears with an otoscope.)

Ms. Kowalsky: She doesn't come when I call her. I have to make my voice loud.

Physician (speaking to the nurse): It's quite red behind this one drum. Looks like otitis media. We caught it early.

Ms. Kowalsky (very alarmed): What's wrong with my Iwona? Otitis? What you talking about?

Nurse (to Ms. Kowalsky): Don't worry Ms. Kowalsky. We'll take care of Iwona. She'll be fine.

Physician (to the nurse): Let's do an audiogram now.

Nurse (to Ms. Kowalsky): Please help Iwona get dressed. I'll be back in a minute to take her for an audiogram.

Ms. Kowalsky was confused. She had no idea what an audiogram was, nor did she understand the term *otitis media*, but she helped Iwona dress. In a few minutes, the nurse returned and led Iwona into another room for the audiogram, leaving the mother to anxiously wait alone.

Nurse (on returning to the room after completing the audio-gram): She (meaning Iwona) had a hard time understanding my directions.

Ms. Kowalsky: My Iwona is very smart. She understands. She knows more words than me. She can tell me the words.

Nurse: According to the audiogram, Iwona doesn't hear sounds the same in both ears. She had trouble telling me what she does hear.

Ms. Kowalsky: My Iwona smart, but she does not hear in her ears good. She tells me "What?" when I tell her come here.

Nurse: I'll show the results to the doctor.

Ms. Kowalsky didn't realize that she should wait to see the doctor (no one explained this to her), so she prepared to leave the clinic.

Physician (stopping the mother in the hallway): I'm giving you a prescription for Iwona's ears. She'll need to swallow medicine four times a day.

Ms. Kowalsky (frustrated and bewildered): Her ears hurt. She have trouble hearing me. How does swallowing pills help her ears?

Physician (harried): Ms. Kowalsky, I wish I had more time to talk with you about Iwona's medication, but I'm really rushed today. When you stop at the pharmacy downstairs, have the pharmacist explain how the medicine works.

Ms. Kowalsky went down to the pharmacy but saw that the waiting room was crowded with patients, all waiting for their prescriptions to be filled. She was exhausted, and Iwona was crying.

Ms. Kowalsky: Come Iwona, we'll go home now. I fix you dinner and we talk to Baba. She'll know what to do for your ears.

Ms. Kowalsky, who did not understand the importance of the antibiotic prescribed by the physician, failed to have the prescription filled. Instead, she relied on the folk medicine remedies recommended by her mother.

Two days later, Iwona's ear infection worsened, and Ms. Kowalsky was forced to return to the clinic with her sick child. The nurse at the clinic blamed Ms. Kowalsky for not giving Iwona the prescribed medicine. In reality, it was the physician's and nurse's responsibility to explain Iwona's illness and its treatment to the mother *in terms she could understand*. For example, the nurse could have said:

> "Ms. Kowalsky, Iwona has an infection in her ears. It's making her ears hurt and it's making it hard for her to hear. We tested her hearing with a procedure called an audiogram. We found that Iwona didn't hear very well in her right ear.
>
> "We need your help to treat Iwona's infection. The doctor wants you to give Iwona an antibiotic medication by mouth, four times a day. The antibiotic will circulate throughout Iwona's system and will fight the infection. It's very important that you give Iwona her medicine on time. Also, you must give her all of the pills the doctor ordered, even when she starts to feel better.
>
> "Do you have any questions? If you think of a question later, call us anytime. We're here to help you."

COMMUNICATION CONSIDERATIONS

To provide optimal care, take the time to explain medical terminology, directions, and procedures to your patients in terms they understand. Encourage patients to ask questions and express feelings and concerns.

OVERCOMING DIFFERENCES IN PERCEPTIONS AND EXPECTATIONS

All nurse–patient communication is to some extent *bicultural*, even when nurse and patient are from the same culture. The patient's **terminology**, **perspective**, **perceptions**, and **expectations** represent the lay culture, whereas the nurse's terminology, perspective, perceptions, and expectations represent the subculture of nursing. When patients and nurses are also from different cultures, communication problems are compounded.

Even when your patients understand medical terminology, their perceptions of illness and health care may be different from yours. These differences can lead to serious misunderstandings during the assessment and treatment process—especially when you are working with patients who adhere to traditional cultural values and behaviors.

Example: On a home visit to the Morales family, a public health nurse found a pair of sharp scissors under the pillow of 4-month-old Anna, and removed them. The nurse, who assumed that Mrs. Morales was being careless, emphatically told the mother to put the scissors away before the infant had an injury. Actually, Mrs. Morales was following an ancient Aztec tradition of leaving needles in the form of a cross under a pillow to ward off evil. Some people who adopted this custom used open scissors (which resemble a cross) in place of needles to keep evil away.

The nurse was surprised when Mrs. Morales began to cry. The nurse responded that Mrs. Morales was crying because she had realized that the scissors might have injured her child. The nurse left the home feeling satisfied that she had prevented an injury. Mrs. Morales, who was angry at the nurse for not respecting her traditions, immediately replaced the scissors under her child's pillow.

In this situation, the nurse would have communicated more effectively with the mother had she asked questions rather than simply assuming that Mrs. Morales was being irresponsible. For instance: "Mrs. Morales, is there some reason that you put scissors under your baby's pillow?" After hearing the mother's explanation, the nurse might add: "I now realize that the scissors have an important meaning for you. However, we don't want your baby to cut herself. Is there a safer item that we can put under the baby's pillow? If not, is there someplace else that we can put the scissors? Do you feel satisfied with this solution?" By acknowledging Mrs. Morales's perception of the scissors and their importance, the nurse could have corrected a potentially hazardous situation without offending and alienating the mother.

Serious misunderstandings also arise when patients *misinterpret* your clinical assessment findings and recommendations. In one case, a nurse in an adolescent clinic told the mother of a 13-year-old boy, "Your son has a positive culture for strep throat. You'll need to bring in your other children right away for throat cultures." The mother (who knew nothing about throat cultures or strep throat) interpreted the nurse's request to mean that she

1. Had neglected her son (who was now ill).

2. Had probably neglected her other children.

3. Must now bring all of her children immediately to the clinic for testing.

Upset and anxious, the mother did not comply with the nurse's recommendation.

To avoid this misunderstanding, the nurse needed to clarify her recommendations as follows: "Your son has strep throat, which can be a very serious infection if it's not treated quickly. This infection spreads easily from person to person. Your other children have been exposed to the germs. Please bring your children in so that we can culture their throats for strep. If your children have strep, we will treat them right away. Let's culture your throat as well. Do you have any questions?"

Different expectations of the nurse's role may also lead to conflicts. For example, patients who use traditional and folk systems of care are not used to a biomedical approach to diagnosis and treatment. They may be suspicious of nurses who perform systematic assessments before giving care and may respond to questions with silence.

Furthermore, some patients may believe that your assessment questions indicate that you lack the knowledge to help them. This problem often arises when assessing patients who are refugees or recent immigrants and who still adhere to traditional beliefs.

Rural Alaskan Natives and Native Americans who have received nursing care only during emergencies (including being driven or airlifted to a hospital) may expect you to rapidly provide care without asking questions, as in an emergency setting. These patients may be reluctant to give a detailed history and to answer questions because they expect a quick assessment.

• • • COMMUNICATION CONSIDERATIONS • • •

To reduce incompatibilities in transcultural communication:

1. Strive to understand the patient's perceptions and expectations of you and the biomedical health care system.

2. Take the time to elicit information about the patient's health care belief system.

3. In simple terms, carefully explain your role in the assessment process and why it is vital that the patient answer your questions.

4. Welcome questions from your patient and answer them as clearly and simply as possible.

5. Allow the patient's traditional healer to visit the hospital; let the patient follow the traditional healing practices, provided that they do not interfere with the prescribed treatment regimen.

6. If the patient's health care practices do conflict with biomedical practices, communicate with your patient until you develop a plan of care that is acceptable to you, the patient, and the physician. Engage in the process of cultural negotiation.

REFERENCES

Agar, M. (1996). *The professional stranger: An informed introduction to ethnography.* New York: Academic Press.

Charonko, D. V. (1992). Cultural influences in noncompliant behavior and decision making. *Holistic Nurse Practitioner, 6*(3), 73–78.

Cherry, B., & Giger, J. N. (1995). African Americans. In: J. N. Giger & R. E. Davidhizar (Eds.), *Transcultural nursing: Assessment and intervention* (2nd ed.). St. Louis: Mosby.

DeSantis, L. (1994). Making anthropology clinically relevant to nursing care. *Journal of Advanced Nursing, 20*(4), 707–715.

Gibbs, R. D., Gibbs, P. H., & Henrich, J. (1987). Patient understanding of commonly used medical vocabulary. *Journal of Family Practice, 25*(2), 176–178.

Stokes, L. G. (1977). Delivering health services in a black community. In A. M. Reinhardt & M. B. Quinn (Eds.), *Current practice in family-centered community nursing.* St. Louis: Mosby.

Urden, L. D., Stacy, K. M., & Lough, M. E. (2001). *Thelan's critical care nursing: Diagnosis and management* (4th ed.). St. Louis: Mosby.

SUGGESTED READINGS

Campinha-Bacote, J. (1995). The quest for cultural competence in nursing care. *Nursing Forum, 30*(4), 19–25.

Cravener, P. (1992). Establishing therapeutic alliance across cultural barriers. *Journal of Psychosocial Nursing, 30*(12), 10–14.

Doswell, W. M. (1998). Multicultural issues and ethical concerns in the delivery of nursing care interventions. *Nursing Clinics of North America, 33*(2), 353–361.

Fairlie, A. (1992). Nurse-patient communication barriers. *Senior Nurse, 12*(3), 40–43.

Fielo, S. B., & Degazon, C. E. (1997). When cultures collide: Decision making in a multicultural environment. *Nursing and Health Care Perspectives, 18*(5), 238–243.

Foong, A. (1992). Challenging the tower of Babel: The increasing diversity in cultures. *Nursing, 5*(5), 12–25.

Giger, J. N., & Davidhizar, R. E. (Eds.). (2003). *Transcultural nursing: Assessment and intervention* (4th ed.). St. Louis: Mosby.

Grossman, D. (1996). Cultural dimensions in home health care. *American Journal of Nursing, 96*(7), 33–36.

Herberg, P. (1995). Theoretical foundations of transcultural nursing. In: M. M. Andrews & J. S. Boyle (Eds.), *Transcultural concepts in nursing care* (2nd ed.). Philadelphia: Lippincott.

Leap, N. (1992). The power of words. *Nursing Times, 88*(21), 60–61.

Leininger, M. (1996). Founder's focus. Transcultural nurses and consumers tell their stories. *Journal of Transcultural Nursing, 7*(2), 32–36.

Newman, J. (1998). Managing cultural diversity: The art of communication. *Radiographic Technology, 69*(3), 231–246, 249.

Purnell, L. D., & Paulanka, B. J. (1998). Purnell's model for cultural competence. In L. D. Purnell & B. J. Paulanka (Eds.), *Transcultural health care: A culturally competent approach*. Philadelphia: Davis.

Purnell, L. D., & Paulanka, B. J. (Eds.). (2003). *Transcultural health care: A culturally competent approach* (2nd ed.). Philadelphia: Davis.

Rothenburger, R. L. (1990). Transcultural nursing: Overcoming obstacles to effective communication. *AORN Journal, 51*(5), 1349–1363.

Sabatino, F. (1993). Culture shock: Are U.S. hospitals ready? *Hospitals, 67*(1), 22–25, 28–31.

Sherer, J. L. (1993). Crossing cultures: Hospitals begin breaking down the barriers to care. *Hospitals, 67*(1), 22–25, 28–31.

Thiederman, S. B. (1986). Ethocentrism: A barrier to effective health care. *Nurse Practitioner, 11*(8), 52–59.

Tips for overcoming cultural barriers. (1998). *Same-Day Surgery, 22*(4), Supplement 4.

Trossman, S. (1998). Diversity: A continuing challenge. *American Nurse, 30*(1), 1, 24–25.

Wright, F., Cohen, S., & Caroselli, C. (1997). Diverse decisions: How culture affects ethical decision making. *Nursing Clinics of North America, 9*(1), 63–74.

CHAPTER 10

Working with and without an Interpreter

KEY TERMS

- Culture Broker
- Equivalent Meaning
- Interpreter
- Language Barrier
- Limited English Proficiency (LEP)
- Office for Civil Rights (OCR)
- Professional Medical Interpreter
- Telephone Interpretation Service
- Translator
- U.S. Department of Health and Human Services (HHS)

OBJECTIVES

After completing this chapter, you should be able to:

- Discuss the role of the medical interpreter, and describe what duties lie within the province of the interpreter's job.
- Differentiate between interpretation and translation.
- List the major provisions of the Code of Ethics for Interpreters in Health Care.
- Identify three vital reasons why medical interpreters are needed in the clinical area, and provide examples of each.
- Discuss a patient's legal right to an interpreter if the patient does not speak English.

- Describe techniques that will help you work successfully with a trained medical interpreter.
- Describe techniques that will help you communicate without the aid of a trained interpreter.

INTRODUCTION

Communicating with patients from different cultures is often complicated by language differences. In the preceding sections on communication, we primarily discussed situations in which the patient and the nurse spoke and understood the same language. Nurses face a far greater challenge when they try to communicate with patients with limited English proficiency or with no proficiency in English. Unless you learn ways to overcome language barriers, your customary assessment and teaching skills will be seriously hampered, and the patient's care may be compromised.

This chapter describes the important role of the medical interpreter and outlines specific techniques for working with and without a medical interpreter when assessing patients and providing care.

WORKING WITH A MEDICAL INTERPRETER

When the patient does not speak English or has limited English proficiency, the best solution is to use a **professional medical interpreter**. These professional interpreters are trained to objectively convey the message without distortions that may result from personal biases, opinions, or experiences. Bilingual proficiency is expected as well as the ability to use appropriate words and jargon that best express the message. To benefit from the services of an interpreter, you should understand exactly what an interpreter does and why a trained or certified interpreter should be used to interpret rather than family members or other unqualified individuals.

The Role of the Medical Interpreter

The Code of Federal Regulations defines a qualified interpreter as "an individual who is able to interpret receptively and expressively, using any necessary specialized vocabulary" (Andrea & Renner, 1996). At a meeting of the National Council on Interpretation in Health Care, attendees agreed that the basic role of the medical interpreter is to facilitate communication between people speaking different languages in a health care setting. Ensuring that people can understand each other is the interpreter's job; the content of what is said is the responsibility of patient and provider (Roat, 1997).

COMMUNICATION CONSIDERATIONS

Sometimes physicians and nurses incorrectly ask interpreters to perform duties that are not a part of their role. For example, it is not appropriate to ask an interpreter to explain diagnoses or procedures or to act as a counselor. Interpreters help with patient assessments and interventions only in that they interpret what the provider and patient are saying to each other. The interpreter should stay in the background unless there is a misunderstanding between patient and provider that the interpreter needs to correct.

A medical interpreter plays a different role than a medical translator. Both interpreters and translators take a concept that is expressed in one language and express it in another language. However, an **interpreter** takes a *spoken* message in one language and renders it in another. A **translator** takes a *written* message in one language and renders it in another; for example, a translator may translate a patient brochure from English to Spanish. Both interpreting and translating are equally accurate, and both relay the denotative (objective) and cognitive (subjective or emotional) meaning of words (Roat, 1997).

Because language reflects a person's reality, experience, culture, and world view, interpreters do not focus on word-to-word equivalence but rather on the accurate expression of **equivalent meaning**. Thus, an experienced interpreter can serve as a **culture broker** and provide a cultural framework for understanding spoken language. That is, an interpreter can convey not only a patient's responses to your questions but also general information about the patient's culture—information that will help in assessment and in planning and implementing care. At the same time, a good interpreter will help the patient understand the biomedical terms you may need to use and the basics of the mainstream health care system. Thus, by linking the two cultures, an interpreter can increase trust and reduce the chances of conflict between nurse and patient.

Some interpreters are better trained as culture brokers than others. Moreover, the health care facilities that employ interpreters may limit what interpreters are allowed to do. Also, understand that interpreters may bring their own biases to a situation. As a result, you may not receive full and accurate information, or the interpreter may provide the patient with information that you did not intend for the patient to receive. Major interpreter biases include (Putsch, 1985):

- Religious, ethnic, and political biases.

- Socioeconomic biases (e.g., a well-educated interpreter or one from an upper-class background may feel inhibited about literally translating patient statements and beliefs that convey folk practices or superstitions).

- Cultural biases (e.g., the interpreter may speak the same language as the patient but may be from a completely different culture).

Because medical interpreting is an emerging field, it does not have a universally accepted code of ethics or training requirements. Roat, an interpreter training coordinator, has written a code of ethics for interpreters in health care that combines codes of ethics from three American health interpretation programs. In order to evaluate your experiences with medical interpreters, familiarize yourself with this code of ethics (Figure 10-1).

A MEDICAL INTERPRETER CODE OF ETHICS

A medical interpreter is a specially trained professional who has proficient knowledge and skills in two languages and employs that training in a health-related setting in order to make possible communication among parties using different languages.

The skills of a medical interpreter include cultural competency and awareness and respect to all parties involved as well as mastery of medical and colloquial terminology, which make possible conditions of mutual trust and accurate communication leading to effective provision of medical/health services.

1. **Confidentiality**

   Interpreters must treat all information learned during the interpretation as confidential, divulging nothing without the full approval of the patient and his or her physician.

2. **Accuracy: conveying the content and spirit of what is said**

   Interpreters must transmit the message in a thorough and faithful manner, omitting or adding nothing, giving consideration to linguistic variations in both languages and conveying the tone and spirit of the original message.

   (continues)

Figure 10-1 Medical Interpreter Code of Ethics *Reprinted with permission of Cynthia E. Roat, MPH, Interpreter Training Coordinator, The Cross-Cultural Health Care Program, PacMed Clinics, Seattle, WA.*

A word-for-word interpretation may not convey the intended idea. The interpreter must determine the relevant concept and say it in language that is readily understandable and culturally appropriate to the person being helped. In addition, the interpreter will make every effort to ensure that the patient has understood questions, instructions and other information transmitted by the health care provider.

3. Completeness: conveying everything that is said

Interpreters must interpret everything that is said by all people in the interaction. If the content to be interpreted might be perceived as offensive, insensitive, or otherwise harmful to the dignity and well-being of the patient, the interpreter should advise the provider of this before interpreting.

4. Conveying cultural frameworks

Interpreters shall explain cultural differences or practices to health care providers and patients when appropriate.

5. Nonjudgmental attitude about the content to be interpreted

An interpreter's function is to facilitate communication. Interpreters are not responsible for what is said by anyone for whom they are interpreting. Even if the interpreter disagrees with what is said or thinks it is wrong or even immoral, the interpreter must suspend judgment, make no comments, and interpret everything accurately.

6. Client self-determination

The interpreter may be asked by the client for his or her opinion. When this happens, the interpreter needs to provide or restate information that will assist the patient in making his or her own decision. The interpreter should not influence the opinion of patients or clients by telling them what action to take.

7. Attitude toward clients

The interpreter should strive to develop a relationship of trust and respect at all times with the patient by adopting a caring, attentive, yet discreet and impartial attitude toward the patient and toward his or her questions, concerns, and needs. The interpreter shall treat each patient equally with dignity and

(continues)

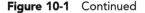

Figure 10-1 Continued

respect regardless of race, color, sex, religion, nationality, political persuasion, or lifestyle choice.

8. Acceptance of assignments

If level of experience or personal sentiments make it difficult to abide by any of the above conditions, the interpreter should decline or withdraw from the assignment.

Interpreters should disclose any real or perceived conflict of interest that would affect their objectivity in delivery of their service. For example, interpreters should refrain from providing services to family members or close personal friends except in emergencies. In personal relationships, it is difficult to remain unbiased or nonjudgmental.

In emergency situations, interpreters may be asked to do interpretations for which they are not qualified. The interpreter may consent only as long as all parties understand the limitations and no other interpreter is available.

9. Compensation

The fee agreed upon by the agency and the interpreter is the only compensation that the interpreter should accept. Interpreters should not accept additional money, considerations, or favors for services reimbursed by the contracting agency. Interpreters should not use the agency's time, facilities, equipment or supplies for private gain or advantage, nor should they use their position to secure privileges or exemptions.

10. Self-evaluation

Interpreters should represent their certification(s), training, and experience accurately and completely.

11. Ethical violations

Interpreters should withdraw immediately from encounters that they perceive to be in violation of the Code of Ethics.

12. Professionalism

Interpreters shall be punctual, prepared, and dressed in an appropriate manner. The trained interpreter is a professional who maintains professional behavior at all times while assisting clients and who seeks to further his or her knowledge and skills through continuing studies and training.

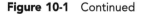

Figure 10-1 Continued

Reasons for Using a Medical Interpreter

There are three major categories of reasons for using a medical interpreter:

1. Legal reasons.
2. Quality of care reasons.
3. Financial reasons.

Legal Reasons. In the 1990 Census, 13.8% of people in the United States spoke a language other than English. Spanish was the most frequently spoken language at home. In some states, percentages of persons speaking another language were higher than the national norm (U.S. Bureau of Census, 1990). Federal laws, as enforced by the **U.S. Department of Health and Human Services (HHS) Office for Civil Rights (OCR)**, state that an individual (or class of individuals) *may not be denied an interpreter* when seeking or receiving treatment at a health care facility that is a recipient of federal funds from HHS. Title VI of the Civil Rights Act of 1964 and its supporting regulations require all health care programs receiving federal funds to provide language assistance to all clients with **limited English proficiency (LEP)**. The Office for Civil Rights Policy Guidelines further stipulate that the use of informal, noncertified interpreters, such as families and friends, is not acceptable as a means of guaranteeing access to services (Office for Civil Rights, 2000). According to the Office for Civil Rights:

> The recipient must have bilingual employees or provide interpreters, translators, and other means to ensure the nondiscriminatory provision of services. Such aids must be provided without additional charge to persons needing them in order to benefit equally from any service, program, or activity.

Furthermore, HHS states, "No person may be subjected to discrimination on the basis of national origin in health and human services programs because they have a primary language other than English" (Perkins, Simon, Cheng, Olson, & Vera, 1998).

In addition to federal laws mandating the use of interpreters in institutions receiving federal funds, some states also require the use of an interpreter whenever a communication barrier exists. For example, the California Health and Safety Code, Section 1259, requires that licensed acute care hospitals "have a policy in effect and provide, to the extent possible, interpreters whenever a communication barrier exists." The Code defines **language barriers** as "barriers experienced by persons who are limited in English speaking or non-English-speaking individuals who speak the same primary language and who comprise at least 5% of the population of the geographic area served by the hospital" (Andrea & Renner, 1996; California Health and Safety Code, 1995).

Unfortunately, although the federal government and many states require hospitals to provide interpreters or risk the loss of government funding, there is still a severe shortage of trained medical interpreters within the nation's health care facilities. First of all, it is difficult to enforce federal and state laws that require hospitals to hire trained interpreters.

In addition, some patients who speak little or no English probably do not know their legal rights and are thus unlikely to file a complaint with government agencies. In an analysis of the legal needs of indigent immigrants, researchers found that obtaining health care was the third most common legal problem. They also learned that very few immigrants with legal problems were able to obtain legal help (Perkins et al., 1998).

Quality of Care Reasons. Many grave problems involving quality of care can arise from miscommunications due to language barriers between patients and health care practitioners. Some of these problems include the following (Fein, 1997):

- Physicians do not receive an accurate history from their patients, and consequently they misdiagnose patients.

- Patients do not understand their medication and treatment schedules and thus fail to follow their treatment regimes.

- Patients agree to procedures and even surgeries without fully understanding the consequences and ramifications of treatment.

- Patients are not aware of and thus fail to seek preventive care.

- Patients, their families, and their health care providers all suffer from severe frustration as they attempt to cross language barriers without the help of a professional interpreter.

•••• COMMUNICATION CONSIDERATIONS ••••

When there is a large immigrant population and not enough skilled interpreters, patient care suffers. Poor patients, in particular, are placed at high risk.

When physicians and nurses are desperate to find someone to interpret for them, they may ask people to interpret who are not qualified. In one southern California hospital, nursing managers reported that "nurses, physicians, students, housekeepers, janitors, clerks, volunteers, patients' friends, and relatives with very little expertise in the language or in medical terminology were relied on to question patients and translate significant medical information" (Rader, 1988). In a large hospital in New York City, an emergency department physician reported being forced to use a Vietnamese restaurant owner to translate over the telephone for his Vietnamese patient (Fein, 1997).

In a study of three hospitals in San Diego, California, emergency department (ED) nurses found that they needed interpreters for 14 languages—Spanish being the most predominant language. The nurses documented that within the ED, 42% of interpreting was done by family members and 33% was done by nonmedical personnel. The family members were often limited in their ability to understand English, and the lay personnel were unable to translate medical terminology correctly. This finding validated the ED's need for trained interpreters with a background in medical terminology (Andrea & Renner, 1996).

COMMUNICATION CONSIDERATIONS

If you are not completely fluent in the patient's language, it is always best to seek the services of a professional interpreter. Patients may be reluctant to let you know that they do not understand what you are saying. Gross misunderstandings between patients and nurses can lead to grave errors in diagnosis and treatment. Use an interpreter when necessary!

Financial Reasons. When interpreters are not available to facilitate communication between non-English-speaking patients and providers, not only does the quality of care decrease, but the *costs* of care increase. Costs can escalate for the following reasons (Perkins et al., 1998):

- Non-English-speaking patients fail to use preventive measures that could prevent costly illnesses and injuries.
- Patients wait to seek medical treatment until their symptoms have worsened, thereby increasing the cost of care.
- Physicians, unable to obtain a full history from the patient, tend to rely on expensive and often unnecessary batteries of tests to make their diagnoses.
- Interventions can take 25% to 50% longer to produce results because non-English-speaking patients may not understand or follow the physician's orders (Hagland, 1993).

- Patients miss crucial appointments with their physicians or nurse practitioners and thus risk suffering unnecessary relapses, which will cost more money to treat.
- Patients may bring malpractice suits or complaints that will be costly and time consuming to address.

COMMUNICATION CONSIDERATIONS

If your health care facility serves a multicultural population and does not employ a trained interpreter, remind administrators that interpreters can both increase the quality and reduce the cost of patient care.

Guidelines for Working with a Medical Interpreter

If you have never worked with a professional interpreter before, you may initially find the process difficult, because you are relying on another person for your collection of verbal data. Remember that clients may not express the need for interpretation, so you need to offer interpreter service. To receive the maximum benefit from the interpreter's services with the least amount of frustration, follow these guidelines:

1. Schedule an interpreter to interpret patient assessment questions and explain instructions for diagnostic and treatment procedures, consent forms, and any other materials and issues that require clear communication.

2. If possible, request an interpreter of the same gender and similar age as the patient. When you are assessing patients from some cultures, especially Asian cultures, it may be more helpful to work with an interpreter who is considerably older than the patient and thus worthy of respect.

3. To make good use of the interpreter's time, decide beforehand on the questions you will ask the patient.

4. Try to communicate with the patient while you are waiting for the interpreter to arrive. Many interpreters suggest that speaking a few words in the patient's language may help the patient relax. Your health care facility may have a phrase chart or picture cards to help you communicate with patients who do not speak English. Even though you may mispronounce words, an attempt on your part to speak the patient's language can help to establish rapport and trust.

•••• COMMUNICATION CONSIDERATIONS ••••

Never ignore patients because they do not speak your language.

5. If possible, meet briefly with the interpreter before you begin your assessment session with the patient. Let the interpreter know what you are planning to ask. If the patient's language does not contain English equivalents for certain symptoms or disorders, work with the interpreter to develop a new line of questioning. For example, the Navajo language does not have an equivalent term for *allergy*. To compensate for the lack of the word *allergy*, you might ask questions to determine whether the patient has had any symptoms of an allergy—such as sneezing, rash, dry mouth, or breathing problems—after taking a medicine.

6. You may want to ask the interpreter for the best way to approach delicate issues such as sexuality, impending death, or informed consent. An experienced interpreter will help you find culturally appropriate ways to ask difficult and personal questions.

7. During the session, face the patient. Sitting protocols for interpreters differ in different parts of the United States. In some areas, interpreters sit beside and a bit behind the patient. Other protocols place the interpreter between the patient and the health care provider, forming a triangle.

8. Direct your questions to the patient and not to the interpreter. Keep appropriate eye contact with the patient when you ask questions and throughout the responses.

9. Remember that even though the patient may not speak English, the person may understand some English. Comments not meant for the patient's ears should be left until the interview is over and you are alone with the interpreter.

10. Talk about one symptom or problem at a time. Do not ask, "Do you have pain, and does it seem to occur when you cough?" Do ask, "Do you have pain?" "Where does it hurt?" "Do you also have a cough?" "Is your cough causing the pain?" Allow the patient sufficient time to answer each question.

11. Use short, concise questions and phrases. Avoid idiomatic expressions or colorful expressions that are culture bound and may confuse the patient. Do not say, "Is this problem a real pain in the neck?" or "Do you have your ups and downs?"

12. Look for changes in the patient's expression when the interpreter is explaining your questions. Avoid becoming so preoccupied with note taking that you forget to assess the patient's tone of voice, body language, and physiologic symptoms such as increased diaphoresis or frequent sighing.

13. If the patient's responses to direct questions are very brief, try a more conversational approach: "Some people tell me this (a symptom) happened to them. Have you had this symptom?"

14. If you think the translated answer is too brief after a lengthy and involved patient answer, ask the interpreter why the answer was so brief. A short answer may be the appropriate interpretation.

15. If the interpreter feels that a question is inappropriate or might offend the patient, wait and discuss the question with the interpreter after the session. Later, the interpreter may find a way to obtain the information you need without offending the patient.

16. Be aware that some interpreters may not always follow the ethical guidelines discussed earlier in this chapter. For instance, they may not convey everything that is being said, they may insert their own ideas, or they may be uncomfortable with the topic of questioning.

17. Listen for new ideas that the patient introduces. With the interpreter's help, try to expand on those ideas. Do not just go through a list of prepared questions.

18. After your assessment session, take a few minutes to review the patient's answers with the interpreter. If the patient seems tired and you have more questions, you and the interpreter may need to schedule a follow-up session.

WORKING WITHOUT A MEDICAL INTERPRETER

Although you should always try to work with a medically trained interpreter, one may not always be available. This section describes (1) how to find someone to temporarily interpret and (2) what you can do to communicate with your patient while you wait for an interpreter to arrive.

Finding Someone Who Can Interpret

When your patient speaks little or no English and a medically trained interpreter is not available, you will need to find someone to interpret for you.

Unfortunately, this complex task tends to fall on the shoulders of anyone who is bilingual and who is readily available—this most often being the patient's family and friends. Although well-meaning, family members and friends are generally not able to interpret precisely and objectively. They may not speak fluent English themselves and usually do not understand medical terminology.

Moreover, in some situations, complications and confusion can arise when family members try to interpret. For example, asking a school-age male family member to interpret for his grandmother may be inappropriate because he may:

1. Be too young to know terms in his native language for certain conditions.

2. Be embarrassed by words his grandmother uses or the beliefs she voices.

3. Not interpret everything you and your patient say.

4. Be put in a difficult position from a cultural standpoint, because interpreting gives him the status normally reserved for the adult head of the household.

COMMUNICATION CONSIDERATIONS

Remember to avoid placing a young family member in the emotional position of interpreting devastating news to an older family member. In this situation, make every effort to find a trained interpreter.

In addition, patients may feel too embarrassed to disclose key information in the presence of their relatives, especially if it is of a delicate or sensitive nature. Then too, relatives may attempt to protect their loved one by correcting the patient's statements to sound more normal. For example, a relative may not tell the nurse that the patient is reporting hallucinations or hearing voices. Also, older children may tend to answer for the patient rather than interpret what the patient actually says, a tendency that results in misleading information and an inaccurate assessment.

Unfortunately, without a professional interpreter, you may be forced to rely on a family member to interpret for the patient, especially before surgery or other procedures and in the postanesthesia recovery room while the patient is regaining consciousness. In emergency situations, you may have little choice but to relay queries through a family member, unless you can find a *bilingual employee* who understands some medical terminology or your health care facility has access to a **telephone interpretation service**.

For example, some health care facilities have an account with the *AT&T Language Line*. This nationwide, 24-hour service provides interpreters for approximately 140 languages. Although this service does not take the place of a trained interpreter at the bedside, it does allow patients who do not speak English to communicate their history and symptoms to health care providers—especially in emergencies.

Because telephone interpreters offer an alternative to having a trained interpreter on staff, they are expensive. Indeed, for small clinics, the cost of this type of service may be prohibitive. Furthermore, the quality of the service varies from interpreter to interpreter. Not all telephone interpreters understand medical terminology. Even those interpreters who do understand medical terms are at a disadvantage, because they are not able to assess verbal and nonverbal clues over the telephone. Finally, some older patients may not want to discuss their symptoms and personal problems with a disembodied voice at the other end of a speakerphone (Andrea & Renner, 1996; Fein, 1997).

Guidelines for Working without an Interpreter

Occasionally, you may not have even a family member or a bilingual employee to interpret for you. What should you do to communicate with your patient while you wait for an interpreter to arrive? (Delk-Calkins, 1984; Puterbaugh, 1991).

If the patient understands a little English, you may be able to gather useful information without an interpreter by following these guidelines:

- Greet the patient respectfully. Be polite and formal, especially with older non-English-speaking patients, Hispanics, and Asians.

- Try to identify your patient's primary language. If you are familiar with any words in this language, use them to show the patient that you are trying to communicate. A simple *buenos dias* or *bonjour* may help to reduce the patient's anxiety level.

- In some situations, you might try a third language in order to communicate. For example, if you speak French, you may be able to communicate with a Vietnamese patient. Because of the French colonial influence in Vietnam, some Vietnamese may be able to speak or read some French. European patients often speak several languages; for example, Polish or Russian patients may also speak French or Spanish. If you took Latin in high school, you may even be able use some Latin terms to communicate with patients who speak the Romance languages (French, Italian, and Spanish), which are based on Latin. For example, the word for *pain* in Latin is *dolor*, in Spanish is *dolor*, and in Italian is *dolari*.

- Speak to the patient slowly, clearly, and quietly in English, if this is your only option. Do not shout. Unfortunately, there is a tendency to treat people who do not understand English as though they are deaf. Make every effort to not appear frustrated, irritated, or hurried.

- As you would if you had an interpreter, talk about one symptom or problem at a time. Use simple sentences, and keep your questions short. Use hand movements as necessary to demonstrate what you are asking. Rather than asking, "Where is the pain and is it sharp or does it throb?" instead, try: "Point out for me the spot where your stomach hurts." "Does it feel like a knife?" "No? Then does it throb?" As you ask these questions, point to your own stomach, or pretend that you are stabbing yourself with a knife.

- Repeat the same question or sentence before restating it in different words.

- Use common, descriptive expressions, and try to avoid using medical terminology. For example, use *bleeding* or *pus* or *liquid* rather than *discharge*.

- Use picture cards or a phrase chart (using phonetic pronunciation) to verify patient information.

- Be aware that some patients may answer yes to all of your questions in order to avoid appearing ignorant or rude. Actually, the patient may have understood very little of what you have tried to say or demonstrate.

Although these techniques may temporarily help you to communicate a little with your patient, it is nonetheless critical that you find an interpreter as quickly as possible—preferably a medically trained interpreter. Check with the nursing office for the names of bilingual employees who understand medical terminology. You might also contact the hospital chaplain or rabbi. These spiritual advisers may speak a foreign language or have contacts with individuals who are proficient in other languages.

REFERENCES

Andrea, J., & Renner, P. (1996). Interpreting the needs of the ED patient: One California hospital's 3 week study. *Emergency Nursing, 21*(6), 510–512.

California Health and Safety Code, Section 1259 (Daring's Supplement, 1995).

Delk-Calkins, K. (1984). What to do until the translator arrives. *Journal of Practical Nursing, 34*(2), 12–13, 61.

Fein, E. B. (1997, November 23). Language barriers are hindering health care. *New York Times*, p. 20.

Hagland, M. M. (1993). Crossing cultures: Hospitals begin breaking down the barriers to care. *Hospitals, 67*, 29.

Office for Civil Rights, HHS (2000). Title VI of the Civil Rights Act of 1964. Policy guidelines on the prohibition against national origin discrimination as it affects persons with limited English proficiency. *Federal Register, 65*(169), 2762–2774.

Perkins, J., Simon, H., Cheng, F., Olson, K., & Vera, Y. (1998). *Ensuring linguistic access in health care settings: Legal rights and responsibilities.* Menlo Park, CA: National Health Law Program for the Henry J. Kaiser Family Foundation.

Puterbaugh, S. (1991). Communicating when the patient cannot speak English. *Today's OR Nurse, 13*(1), 31.

Putsch, R. W. (1985). Cross-cultural communication: The special case of interpreters in health care. *Journal of the American Medical Association, 254*(23), 3344–3348.

Rader, G. S. (1988, July). Management decisions: Do we really need interpreters? *Nursing Management, 19*(7), 46–48.

Roat, C. E. (1997). A medical interpreter's code of ethics. In C. E. Roat (Ed.), *Bridging the gap: A basic training for medical interpreters: Trainer's curriculum* (pp. 34–35). Seattle, WA: Cross-Cultural Health Care Program.

U.S. Bureau of Census. (1990). Washington, DC: Government Printing Office. November, 1992.

SUGGESTED READINGS

Andrews, M. M., & Boyle, J. S. (2003). *Transcultural concepts in nursing care* (4th ed.). Philadelphia: Lippincott.

Dinh, H. (1997). Translation initiative. *Contemporary Nurse, 6*(2), 75–76.

Giger, J. N., & Davidhizar, R. E. (Eds.). (1999). *Transcultural nursing: Assessment and intervention* (3rd ed.). St. Louis: Mosby.

Haffner, L. (1992). Translation is not enough: Interpreting in the medical setting. (Cross-cultural medicine—A decade later). *Western Journal of Medicine, 157* (Special issue), 255–259.

Hatton, D. C. (1992). Information transmission in bilingual, bicultural contexts. *Journal of Community Health Nursing, 9*(1), 53–59.

Hatton, D. C. (1993). Information transmission in bilingual, bicultural contexts: A field study of community health nurses and interpreters. *Journal of Community Health Nursing, 10*(3), 137–147.

Kaufert, J. M. (1997). Communication through interpreters in healthcare: Ethical dilemmas arising from differences in class, culture, language, and power. *Journal of Clinical Ethics, 8*(1), 71–87.

Newman, J. (1998). Managing cultural diversity: The art of communication. *Radiographic Technology, 69*(3), 231–246, 249.

Purnell, L. D., & Paulanka, B. J. (1998). *Transcultural health care: A culturally competent approach*. Philadelphia: Davis.

Title 45 Code of Federal Regulations, Part 80—Nondiscrimination under programs receiving federal assistance through the Department of Health and Human Services effectuation of Title VI of the Civil Rights Act of 1964. Department of Health and Human Services, 45 CFRA (10-1-94 Edition), pp. 292–293.

Woloshin, S., & Bickell, N. A. (1995) Language barriers in medicine in the United States. *Journal of the American Medical Association, 273*(9), 724–728.

UNIT TWO
EVALUATION

EVALUATING YOUR
TRANSCULTURAL COMMUNICATION SKILLS

Exercise One: Evaluating How Comfortable You Feel When Communicating with Patients from Other Cultures

Recall that you performed this exercise before you started Unit Two. By now you should have read all of the chapters in the unit. Also, you probably have had an opportunity to visit at least one ethnic community and take care of several patients from different cultures. The statements that follow contain assignments that you may have received in the clinical area or community. Using the five levels of comfort, rate how comfortable you *now* feel about performing each assignment. Compare your current levels of comfort with your earlier levels.

- Level 1: I feel very uncomfortable.
- Level 2: I feel rather uncomfortable.
- Level 3: I feel fairly comfortable.
- Level 4: I feel comfortable.
- Level 5: I feel very comfortable.

1. *Assignment:* Go into a market in an ethnic neighborhood and ask the store personnel about the different foods that are available and how to prepare them.   **1 2 3 4 5**

2. *Assignment:* Go to an ethnic pharmacy and speak with the pharmacist about which over-the-counter drugs the people in the neighborhood tend to purchase.   **1 2 3 4 5**

3. *Assignment:* Visit a cuandero or folk healer and learn about the various healing modalities that he or she uses.   **1 2 3 4 5**

4. *Assignment:* Admit an older Asian female patient who is accompanied by many concerned, attentive family members.   **1 2 3 4 5**

5. *Assignment:* Admit an Italian patient who is constantly crying and grabbing onto your hand.   **1 2 3 4 5**

6. *Assignment:* Provide home care to a 4-month-old child whose mother has placed open scissors (resembling a cross) under the child's pillow in order to ward off evil spirits. **1 2 3 4 5**

7. *Assignment:* Give a complete bath to a Vietnamese woman with the husband and older children present throughout the procedure.

   1 2 3 4 5

8. *Assignment:* Have a medical interpreter help you collect verbal data from a patient who does not speak English. **1 2 3 4 5**

9. *Assignment:* Admit a patient who does not speak English without the help of an interpreter. **1 2 3 4 5**

Exercise Two: Assessing Your Point of View toward Transcultural Nursing Situations

You also performed this exercise earlier in the self-assessment section of this unit. Select the one answer that best describes your point of view *now* that you have completed the unit. There is no scoring for these questions.

1. The nurse in the nurse–patient interaction needs to
   a. elicit the patient's perspective about being ill
   b. share food with the patient
   c. adopt the patient's customs
   d. efficiently manage the care of the patient

2. A culturally sensitive nurse
   a. is knowledgeable about cultural traits
   b. adheres to institutional regulations
   c. adapts communication style to be congruent with the patient's expectations
   d. develops expertise in asking questions to gather patient data

3. The attention that should be allotted to communication in transcultural settings is
   a. little or none, because few instances are truly cultural exchanges
   b. fairly significant because many patients are from diverse cultural backgrounds
   c. of consequence only in some settings
   d. extremely important and necessary for holistic nursing care

4. When working with a patient in the emergency room who has limited English proficiency, I would
   a. have a close family member interpret for the patient
   b. rely on a telephone language service for pertinent information
   c. make an effort to find a qualified interpreter
   d. attempt to communicate with the patient using a phrase chart

5. When interacting with patients, I would
   a. encourage them to express their views of illness
   b. discourage personal beliefs, because they have little connection to the health care plan
   c. elicit information about their family
   d. insist that they need to comply with their care plan for their own good

Exercise Three: Reviewing Your *Transcultural Interaction Diary*

1. Have you had an opportunity to interact with members of an ethnic community? _____ Who were the individuals you interacted with?

   What did you learn about the culture from each of your interactions?

2. Have you succeeded in developing a therapeutic relationship with a patient from another culture? _____

   What techniques did you use to establish communication with this patient? _____

   Are there other techniques that you might have used to establish communication? _____

   Did you use a process recording format to record your interactions?

   Did you find that format helpful? _____

3. Did you work on overcoming one transcultural communication barrier every week? _____ Which barriers did you focus on?

How successful have you been in identifying and overcoming these barriers? _____

4. Have you had an opportunity to work with an interpreter? _____

What techniques did you use to facilitate your interaction with the patient and the interpreter? _____

_____

Are there any other techniques that you plan to try during future patient–interpreter sessions?

_____

_____

_____

_____

Exercise Four: Evaluating Your Knowledge of Basic Transcultural Communication Techniques

Write a brief response to these questions, which are drawn from topics discussed in Chapters 7 through 10.

1. All repetitive social situations (RSSs) occur in a *context*. What is a context, and why is context forever changing? _____

_____

_____

_____

2. When nurses act as participant-observers, they should try to do the following (give *one example* of each activity, and note if you have participated in this activity):

a. Overcome selective inattention:

_____

b. Use wide-angle lenses:

_____

c. Be both an insider and an outsider:

_____

d. Be introspective:

_____

e. Interview people:

_____

f. Keep field notes:

_____

3. When one is acting as a *complete observer*, the four methods for gathering basic information about cultural groups are:

   a. _____

   b. _____

   c. _____

   d. _____

4. What are the two general methods for being an *observer as participant*? Give examples of each method.

   a. _____

   b. _____

5. What is the difference between a therapeutic relationship and a friendship? _____

6. List three techniques you can use to establish rapport with patients from other cultures.

   a. _____

   b. _____

   c. _____

7. What communication techniques would you use to learn more about a patient who is a recent refugee and a victim of torture? _____

   _____

   _____

8. What techniques can you use to respond to a patient's silence?

   a. _____

   b. _____

   c. _____

   d. _____

9. For each of the following transcultural barriers, give an example of the barrier and a technique for overcoming it.

   a. *Knowledge deficit:*

   Example _____

   Technique _____

   b. *Bias:*

   Example _____

   Technique _____

   c. *Stereotyping:*

   Example _____

   Technique _____

    d. *Terminology differences:*
       Example _____
       Technique _____
    e. *Differences in perceptions and expectations:*
       Example _____
       Technique _____

10. Language barriers can bring a halt to transcultural communication. To overcome language barriers, it is always best to secure the services of a medical interpreter. The difference between translating and interpreting is: _____

   _____

11. What are the three interpreting styles?
    a. _____
    b. _____
    c. _____

12. If you wanted to assess a patient's symptoms, what would you ask the interpreter? _____

   _____

   _____

13. If an interpreter were not immediately available, what are two means of acquiring patient data?
    a. _____
    b. _____

UNIT THREE

Using Transcultural Communication to Elicit Assessment Data and Develop Nursing Diagnoses

UNIT THREE
ASSESSMENT

ASSESSING YOUR ABILITY TO ELICIT ASSESSMENT DATA AND DEVELOP NURSING DIAGNOSES

Exercise One: Assessing Your Personal Objectives

Now that you have studied the basics of transcultural communication in Units One and Two, it is important to set some new personal objectives. What do you want to gain from studying this unit? Check the points in the following list that apply to you. Also, write down any other personal objectives.

My personal objectives are to:

_____ Learn how to perform a cultural assessment.

_____ Overcome the barrier of cultural blind spot syndrome.

_____ Identify my patients' cultural preferences: for instance, what foods they prefer or religious rituals they wish to observe.

_____ Elicit my patients' explanations for their illnesses.

_____ Learn about my patients' patterns of seeking help for their problems.

_____ Feel comfortable when asking a patient's family and friends for information.

_____ Learn how to identify nursing diagnoses that may be culturally biased.

_____ Increase my skill in developing nursing diagnoses for culturally diverse patients.

_____ Develop specific strategies for communicating culturally appropriate nursing diagnoses to other health care professionals.

My other personal objectives for learning how to assess culturally diverse patients and develop appropriate nursing diagnoses are to:

1. _____

2. _____

3. _____

4. _____

5. _____

Exercise Two: Assessing Your Personal Responses to Performing Assessments and Developing Nursing Diagnoses

More and more of the patients we care for come from cultures other than our own. These patients and their families depend on us to accurately *assess* and *identify health problems and concerns.* How *competent* do you really feel when performing these vital activities? Please take a minute to answer the following questions. You will not need to share these answers with anyone, so try to be honest with yourself.

	Agree	Neutral	Disagree
I should be able to learn how to perform a competent cultural assessment within a few months.	_____	_____	_____
I do not need to culturally assess a patient from my own culture.	_____	_____	_____
I need to ask my patients what they believe has caused their illness.	_____	_____	_____
I think that most people do self-care before seeking medical care.	_____	_____	_____
I am comfortable writing nursing diagnoses for patients from other cultures.	_____	_____	_____
I understand how to use nursing diagnoses.	_____	_____	_____
When writing nursing diagnoses, I frequently ask myself: Could I be wrong?	_____	_____	_____
I believe that writing nursing diagnoses is a waste of time.	_____	_____	_____
Some of the nursing diagnoses I have used do not seem to make any sense.	_____	_____	_____
Patients should be involved in their nursing diagnoses and treatment.	_____	_____	_____
Nursing diagnoses must be applied equally to every patient, regardless of culture.	_____	_____	_____

Exercise Three: Using Your *Transcultural Interaction Diary*

1. Before you begin this unit, please set up two new sections in your *Transcultural Interaction Diary*. Devote one section to your experiences, thoughts, and feelings when performing cultural assessments. Use the other section for recording and analyzing your progress as you develop nursing diagnoses for patients from different cultures.

2. Start working with your diary now, before studying this unit.

3. Before reading Chapter 11, think about the patient assessments that you have performed in the past. Were you aware of the vital cultural component that should be a part of all patient assessments? Did you ask your patients about their cultural preferences or their views of illness? Did you feel comfortable inquiring about your patients' cultural backgrounds?

4. Before reading Chapter 12, recall nursing diagnoses that you have written in the past for patients from diverse cultures. Was the experience of writing these nursing diagnoses positive, neutral, or negative? Did you find the NANDA nursing diagnosis list to be helpful or confusing?

5. As you study this unit, use your diary to record the assessments you perform and the nursing diagnoses that you develop for people from different cultures. For each nursing diagnosis, document the assessments (defining characteristics) you identified as supporting that diagnosis. Write down your thoughts, beliefs, and feelings concerning your assessments and diagnoses. Document how you researched and validated each nursing diagnosis before using it in a care plan.

6. Continue to keep your diary as you reflect on the information in this unit. Use the suggested techniques presented in each chapter for improving your ability to assess patients and identify culturally appropriate nursing diagnoses. Note how using a particular nursing diagnosis can help or hinder transcultural communication between you, your patient, and your patient's family.

CHAPTER 11

Eliciting Assessment Data from the Patient, Family, and Interpreters

KEY TERMS

- Cultural Assessment
- Cultural Blind Spot Syndrome
- Cultural Skill
- Cyclical Pattern of Seeking Help
- Dreyfus Model of Skill Acquisition

- Ethnic Elder
- Explanatory Model
- Family Liaison
- Family Survey
- Fong's CONFHER Model
- Genogram
- Linear Pattern of Seeking Help

OBJECTIVES

After completing this chapter, you should be able to:

- Identify questions that you might ask patients to determine their cultural background and preferences.
- Identify and ask questions that will elicit the patient's perspective on illness (explanatory model) as well as the family's viewpoints.
- Identify patterns patients use when seeking help.
- Select the important steps you should initially take when eliciting information from the patient's family.

- Use various subtle communication approaches when routine elicitation techniques are not effective.
- Culturally assess your patients who are ethnic elders.

INTRODUCTION

Broadly defined, a **cultural**, or *culturological*, **assessment** is "a systematic appraisal or examination of individuals, groups, and communities as to their cultural beliefs, values, and practices to determine explicit needs and intervention practices within the cultural context of the people being evaluated" (Leininger, 1978). The cultural assessment is vitally important because it helps to ensure that health care providers will (1) understand and respect each patient's cultural beliefs, values, and practices and (2) take these cultural factors into account when developing a plan of treatment. In support of the cultural assessment, the Joint Commission on Accrediation of Health Care Organizations has concluded that "the impact of the person's culture is an important component of the assessment process" (Terrance, 1994).

The nurse also needs to consider the level of acculturation of the patient. Some individuals from another culture may be very assimilated into the mainstream American culture. Others may be bicultural and hold values of both the majority and the minority groups. Some persons may have been born in the United States but have distinct physical characteristics attributable to their ethnicity such as physical stature, skin color, or shape of the eyes; making assumptions about individuals on the basis of physical appearance may lead to inaccurate conclusions about the patient.

• • • COMMUNICATION CONSIDERATIONS • • •

Remember to do cultural assessments on all patients, including those who are from the same culture as you are. Every patient has beliefs and values that are based on culture, and every patient is entitled to a cultural assessment. If you fail to conduct a cultural assessment simply because the patient is from the same background as you are, you may be falling into the trap of "cultural blind spot syndrome" (Campinha-Bacote, 1995).

Recall from Chapter 5 that **cultural blind spot syndrome** is the belief that "Just because the client looks and behaves much the way you do, you assume that there are no cultural differences or potential barriers to care" (Buchwald, Caralis, & Gany, 1994). For instance, if you are a white nurse and you are assigned a white patient, you may incorrectly assume that you do not need to inquire about this patient's cultural preferences and beliefs because you are both white. Although white Americans may have many cultural values in common, white Americans also come from a vast array of cultural and religious backgrounds: for example English, Irish, German, French, Amish, and Appalachian backgrounds. To avoid cultural blind spot syndrome, you will need to learn as much about the cultural backgrounds and preferences of your white patients as you learn about your nonwhite patients.

This chapter will teach you techniques for eliciting information about your patients' (1) cultural backgrounds and preferences, (2) viewpoints concerning illness, and (3) patterns of seeking medical help. This chapter also discusses how to elicit cultural information from the patient's family and friends and how to culturally assess elders from different ethnic backgrounds.

THE ART OF ELICITING INFORMATION

Conducting a successful cultural assessment is an art and a skill that demands knowledge, patience, creativity, and years of practice. **Cultural skill** is the ability to assess patients' cultural beliefs and preferences. In the process of learning how to conduct a detailed cultural assessment, nurses seem to pass through five distinct stages before they become experts. The following five levels of experience are based on a modified version of the **Dreyfus Model of Skill Acquisition**, which was originally used to study chess players and airline pilots and later was adapted for nurses (Benner, 1984; Campinha-Bacote, 1995; Dreyfus & Dreyfus, 1980).

Level One

Novice nurses have very little cultural skill. They know that they should conduct a cultural assessment, but they do not know how to do so effectively. Novices may feel uncomfortable asking patients what they feel are personal questions. Also, they may fear being viewed by patients as racist. To rise to the next level, novice nurses must face and overcome their feelings of discomfort, learn more about the different cultures with which they have contact, observe how experienced nurses conduct a cultural assessment, and find a mentor to help them.

Level Two

Advanced beginning nurses are able to conduct a marginally acceptable cultural assessment. By this point, these nurses are more culturally conscious than they were as novices. They have attended classes on assessment and are familiar with the different assessment tools. However, because they still lack experience, they do everything according to the rules. Advanced beginning nurses are afraid to deviate from an assessment tool, and they still lack the skills to think critically and creatively while conducting a cultural assessment.

Level Three

Culturally competent nurses usually have two to three years of experience in performing cultural assessments with patients from diverse cultures. Nurses who have achieved cultural competency are able to differentiate between important and irrelevant information. They also are more creative in their approach to asking questions, and they no longer need to rely completely on a cultural assessment tool when conducting an interview. However, competent nurses are not as confident or as flexible as proficient nurses.

Level Four

Proficient nurses have between three and five years of experience conducting cultural assessments. Nurses at this level are able to evaluate the information they learn from patients in a holistic manner. For example, a novice nurse might view patient noncompliance as a negative attitude that must be corrected. A proficient nurse would recognize that the patient is not necessarily being uncooperative but is simply adhering to cultural beliefs and remedies that differ from those prescribed by the biomedical health care system.

Level Five

Expert nurses are so experienced in performing cultural assessments that they no longer need to rely on specific rules or assessment tools. Because they have interviewed hundreds of patients from different cultures, these nurses are able to *intuit* what questions they should ask, and they know how to seek information in a sensitive manner. Expert nurses know what feels right without consciously thinking about what they should ask. To develop their intuitive powers, expert nurses must dedicate many years to learning the art of eliciting cultural information from patients and developing accurate cultural profiles.

ELICITING BASIC CULTURAL INFORMATION

To develop a cultural profile of your patient that you can use when planning care, you will need to conduct a thorough cultural assessment. As you ask questions to determine the patient's cultural background, values, and current needs and preferences, remember to use the basic transcultural communication techniques that are presented in Chapter 9. Also, to facilitate the assessment process, your health care facility may have a checklist that includes items for patients' preferences in diet, personal care, religious beliefs, and so forth. If it does not have one, the Cultural Assessment Questionnaire (Figure 11-1) contains sample questions.

The material presented in this figure is partially based on **Fong's CONFHER model**, which provides a systematic framework for organizing your cultural assessment questions and answers. CONFHER stands for the person's Communication style, Orientation, Nutrition, Family relationships, Health beliefs, Education, and Religion (Fong, 1985). In addition to these categories, the Cultural Assessment Questionnaire contains sections of questions concerning occupational and socioeconomic status, personal care, and hospital experiences (Rosenbaum, 1991).

CULTURAL ASSESSMENT QUESTIONNAIRE

1. **Communication**
   - Do you speak English as your primary language?
   - Do you speak another language at home?
   - Do you read English? Do you read another language?
   - Do you understand common medical terms such as *pain*, *fever*, and *nausea*?
   - Is there a family member to interpret when the hospital (agency) interpreter may not be available?

2. **Orientation or cultural affiliation**
   - Where were you born?
   - How long have you lived in the United States?
   - Were your parents born in the United States?
   - How long have your parents lived in the United States?
   - Do you or your parents still follow the traditions of your native land (or culture)?

3. **Nutrition**
   - Do you prefer certain foods (vegetarian diet, diet free from pork)?
   - Should food be prepared in a certain way (no fried foods)?
   - Do you want family members to bring in specific foods?
   - Do you abstain from any foods? Do you abstain for religious reasons or for health reasons?
   - How often do you prefer to eat?
   - With whom do you usually share your meals?
   - What utensils do you prefer to use?
   - Are there any foods or drinks that help you to feel better when you are ill?

(continues)

Figure 11-1 Cultural Assessment Questionnaire

4. **Family relationships**
   - Who are the members of your immediate or nuclear family?
   - Do you have extended family—in other words, aunts, uncles, cousins, nephews, nieces?
   - Who is the head of your household?
   - Who manages the financial matters within your household?
   - Where do you and your family live? In the city, the suburbs, or a rural area?
   - What do you and your family do together for recreation?
   - Do you have family members who will be visiting you in the hospital?
   - How will family members help you during your hospitalization (being present, doing certain things for you)?
   - Who will take over your duties at home while you are in the hospital?

5. **Health beliefs**
   - What do you do to stay healthy?
   - What do you feel is a healthy diet? Do you try to follow this diet?
   - What do you do for exercise?
   - Is there anything else that you do to stay healthy?
   - Except for this current illness, do you feel that you are reasonably healthy?
   - What do you think are the major reasons people become ill?
   - Why do you think you have become ill?

6. **Educational background**
   - What is the last grade or degree that you completed in school?
   - Did you go to school primarily in the United States? If not, where did you go to school?
   - Are there any subjects that you have studied outside of school?
   - Are you or your family acquainted with medical terminology?
   - Do you learn best from written materials, audiovisual materials, or a hands-on approach?

7. **Religious affiliation**
   - Do you have religious objects (Bible, amulets) that you want to keep at your bedside?
   - Do you belong to a church group or other religious affiliation?
   - Do you wear clothing with a religious significance (prayer shawl, garment, or cross)?
   - Do you normally pray at certain times during the day?
   - Do you observe the Sabbath or any upcoming religious holidays?
   - Are there any spiritual practices that help you feel better (prayer, meditation, reading scriptures, watching religious programs on television)?

(continues)

Figure 11-1 Continued

- Would you like a visit from a representative of your religion?
- Do you consult a religious healer?
- Does your religious faith restrict any specific food or drink?
- Do you fast or refrain from eating certain foods at certain times of the day, week, or month?
- Are you excused from fasting when ill?

8. **Occupation and socioeconomic status**
   - What type of work do you do?
   - Does anyone else in your family work?
   - Do you or your spouse have benefits such as health and dental insurance?
   - Do you receive paid sick days, and if so, how many per year?

9. **Hospital experiences**
   - Have you ever been hospitalized before?
   - When were you hospitalized?
   - Where were you hospitalized?
   - What was your hospitalization like?
   - Is there anything I can do to make this hospitalization easier for you?

10. **Personal care**
    - Do you prefer to bathe in the morning or in the evening?
    - Should the nurse follow any special order or routine?
    - Do you prefer a family member to assist with your personal care?
    - Do you prefer to do as much of your personal care as possible?

Figure 11-1 Continued

Sometimes it may be difficult to obtain this valuable personal and cultural data from a patient during an initial interview. For example, if the person is admitted with severe chest pain and shortness of breath, you will need to obtain most of the preliminary information from the patient's family or friends and then plan to interview the patient later.

Furthermore, you may not be able to conduct an accurate assessment because of language differences. The use of a professionally medically trained interpreter is mandated by law when the patient has limited English proficiency. Use of children and other family members is not encouraged because personal and sensitive information may not be shared through the family member. Chapter 10 describes the techniques that you should use when working with and without an interpreter.

It may also be difficult to obtain complete and accurate cultural information from elderly patients. It may be difficult to interview elderly patients because they may not see or hear well, and some may not own glasses or a hearing aid. Also, ethnic elders may fear your ridicule if they speak honestly about their cultural values and beliefs. To obtain important cultural information from older patients, take care to:

1. Show respect. Always address your elderly patients by their last name unless they give you permission to use their first name or a nickname.

2. Use a trained interpreter if the patient speaks little English.

3. Provide the patient with glasses, a hearing aid, or a pocket talker if needed.

4. Interview the patient in a quiet setting and provide optimum lighting.

5. Smile and show that you are interested in the patient's comfort. For example, provide a warm blanket or a cool beverage.

6. Encourage the patient to talk with you about any fears linked to hospitalization or treatment.

7. Ask the patient if he or she is taking any medicinal herb or receiving treatment from indigenous healers.

8. If the patient sees a traditional healer for health problems, ask if the patient would like you to call this person and arrange for a visit.

• • • COMMUNICATION CONSIDERATIONS • • •

When obtaining a medical history from ethnic elders, health practitioners frequently neglect doing a cultural assessment (Evans & Cunningham, 1996).

In addition to these general cultural assessment guidelines, bear in mind the following special precautions:

• Avoid asking a female patient from a Far Eastern culture about her reproductive history and related issues in the presence of males. Similarly, a Hispanic woman's modesty may make her hesitant to discuss reproductive or genitourinary concerns with her children present.

- Recognize that in some cultures, including Ethiopian culture, women are socialized to be fragile. You may need to obtain information through a woman's husband or a close male family friend.

- When assessing a Native American patient, do not initially ask questions in a rapid manner. Try a gentler, slower approach. First, identify yourself and then state your name, position, and how long you have worked in the agency or facility. Next, tell the patient and family what you hope to do, and then ask questions. Shake hands at the end, not at the beginning, of your meeting.

- Keep in mind that in some cultures, the elder or a male member of the family is expected to respond to questions and make decisions for the patient.

ELICITING VIEWS OF ILLNESS USING THE EXPLANATORY MODEL

The **explanatory model** (EM), a term used by anthropologists, is the patient's explanation for why an illness developed and conception of how the illness should be treated. The EM interview "is designed to elicit a patient's personal, family, social, and cultural beliefs about health, etiology of the illness, onset of symptoms, pathophysiology, course of the illness, and treatment" (Mauksch & Roesler, 1990). Compared with patients who are simply told what to do, patients who are encouraged to discuss their perceptions of illness and expectations for treatment: (1) experience a greater sense of control and feel more involved in their own care, (2) suffer less from anxiety, and (3) are more likely to accept hospital routines and treatment schedules. In sum, patients feel less like powerless pawns that medical personnel push about at random and more like active members of the health care team.

On the other hand, patients who do not accept the biomedical health care system may hesitate to express health beliefs that are unorthodox or based on folk medicine for fear of ridicule from their nurse or physician. For example, patients who explain illness on the basis of a belief that supernatural forces cause the illness or distress may not readily reveal this belief to the health care provider. For this reason, it is very important to ask questions in a sensitive, unhurried way and to express your respect for the patient's viewpoint (Jackson, 1993).

As you assess patients, choose questions that will help you decipher what your patients believe about their current illness (Germain, 1992). For example:

- What do you feel caused your illness?

- When and how did your illness begin?
- Why do you think it started when it did?
- How has this illness affected you physically? How has it affected you mentally? Do you feel upset about being ill?
- Has the illness interfered with your job or forced you to change your lifestyle? What course has your illness taken?
- Do you feel ill all of the time? Do you sometimes feel better and then have another attack?
- How do you think your illness should be treated?
- What do you think we can do to treat your illness? What are your expectations?
- Do you think that your illness is curable?

• • • COMMUNICATION CONSIDERATIONS • • •

Remember that the concern in your voice is more important than the exact way you word a question.

To further clarify your patients' views, incorporate at least some of the following questions (based on questions asked by admissions nurses and nurses who triage patients in emergency rooms) into your assessment:

- What do you call this problem you are having? *Note:* Listen to the patient's term and use that term instead of *it* in the following questions.
- When did *it* start and why do you think *it* started when *it* did?
- What problems has *it* brought into your life?
- What problems has *it* caused your family?
- Why do you think that *it* has affected this particular part of your body?
- Why do you think *it* happened to you and not to someone else?
- What have you done to feel better?
- Have you done anything else to feel better?
- Why are you seeking our help to treat *it* now?
- What would you like us to do to help you recover from *it*?
- Are there any other people who are helping you with your problem?

All of these questions may be modified if you are talking to a *parent* or to a *family member* of the patient:

- Why did you bring (patient's name) to the office, ER, clinic?
- What problem does (patient's name) have that concerns you?
- When did (use the term for the illness supplied by the family, represented here by *it*) start?
- Why do you think *it* started when *it* did?
- Have you done anything to help (patient's name) feel better?
- Has anyone else treated (patient's name)?
- What do you hope we can do for (patient's name)?

Some patients may decide to not answer any of your questions because terrifying past experiences have made them afraid to talk openly with people in authority. For example, refugee survivors of torture may be reluctant to talk with you about their experiences because they may feel that you will not believe them, or they may be ashamed to talk about what their captors did to them (Chester & Holtan, 1992). In such cases, you might want to try the *indirect approach*:

1. Discuss the problems reported by other patients with similar symptoms or with the same illness. For example: "Patients who have the same symptoms as you tell me that they also can't sleep. Have you had problems sleeping?"

2. Change a question into a narrative statement. "My patients tell me they sometimes forget to take their medicines. Do you sometimes forget?"

3. Ask if they use a special term to apply to a problem. For example, "Does your language have a term for acute anxiety?" This form of question appeals to your patient's cultural beliefs and seems less direct than asking about a personal problem.

4. Ask the patient about his or her general knowledge of a situation rather than specifics. For instance, "I recently read about the harsh treatment of political prisoners in your country. Can you tell me more about this situation?"

5. Use additional questions that focus on family knowledge. For example, "Do any of your family members know what to do to help you with your problem? What has worked for you and your family in the past?"

Levin, Like, and Gottlieb (2000) developed a framework for culturally competent clinical practice called ETHIC. This framework can be used as a guide for determining questions for the nursing assessment and providing care.

   E. *Explanation.* To elicit information about the illness, ask the following questions:

   - What do you think may be the reason you have these symptoms?
   - What do friends, family, others say about these symptoms?
   - Have you heard about this illness?
   - Did you read about it in a magazine or newspaper? See or hear about it on television or radio?

   T. *Treatment.* To elicit information about the patient's views on treatment, ask the following questions:

   - What kinds of medicines, home remedies, or other treatments have you tried for this illness?
   - Is there anything you eat, drink, or do (or avoid) on a regular basis to stay healthy? Tell me about it.
   - What kind of treatment are you seeking from me?

   H. *Healers.* To determine the patient's sources of health information, ask:

   - Have you gotten any advice from alternative healers, friends, or other people (nondoctors) for help with your problem? Tell me about it.

   I. *Intervention.* Determine an intervention with your patient.

   C. *Collaboration.* Collaborate with the patient, family, other health care team members, healers, and community resources.

ELICITING THE PATIENT'S PATTERN OF SEEKING HELP

Recall from our earlier discussions that people from different cultures rely on a variety of methods for seeking medical help. Patients may seek help from the popular sector, including:

- Asking advice from family and friends.
- Buying over-the-counter remedies.
- Preparing special diets.
- Participating in exercise programs or practicing meditation or both.

For example, when ill, immigrant patients and patients from refugee groups typically turn first to close family members for help and go to the unfamiliar biomedical care system only as a last resort. People also seek help from such traditional healers as spiritualists, acupuncturists, and curanderos. These traditional healers are esteemed within their culture and are recognized for their diagnostic and treatment skills.

Patients from different cultures often seek help from more than one source. According to some cultural beliefs, biomedical healers are able to treat the immediate cause of illness but not the ultimate cause. For this reason, some patients may use the emergency department for an acute injury but visit a spiritualist or acupuncturist for chronic, lingering symptoms.

Patients often use treatment sources in a **linear pattern**—first asking advice from a friend or family member, then going to a biomedical care facility, and then to a traditional healer such as a religious person, a curandero, a spiritualist, or an acupuncturist. Alternatively, patients may follow a **cyclical pattern** of initially seeking biomedical care, then using a traditional healer, and finally returning to the biomedical care system.

Consider the following pattern of care seeking that involves the use of *multiple sources of care*. Migrant farm workers in California may treat themselves with different available remedies and wait until they have a life-threatening infection or other disabling condition before seeking biomedical health care. Resorting to biomedical care may be late in the patient's pattern of health care seeking because (1) workers must depend on their hourly wage to support their families; (2) workers may have limited or no access to affordable health care; and (3) workers usually rely on time-honored alternative treatments that have been transmitted from one generation to another (Jezewski, 1990).

In a study of the use of multiple sources of care, researchers interviewed a group of 203 blacks with hypertension (high blood pressure). These individuals initially tried to let their bodies heal through prayer or traditional approaches, such as swallowing a pinch of garlic after eating or drinking sassafras tea and lemon juice. Next, the individuals evaluated daily activities, sought advice from a family member, and, last, sought medical assistance (Bailey, 1991).

To assess which methods your patients use for seeking help, ask the following questions (Bushy, 1992):

- Have you done anything to treat the problem?

- What do you do to relieve your discomfort? Does anything you do make you feel better? Is there anything else you do?

- Is there anyone you ask for advice?

- Is there anyone you go to for care besides your medical doctor? Do you seek care from a practitioner, healer, extended family member, or neighbor who is not a medical doctor? Would you like us to contact this person?

- Do you ever go to the drugstore or health food store for remedies you can buy over the counter?

- Do you ever try medicines that your family or friends give you?

COMMUNICATION CONSIDERATIONS

A large portion of patients do self-care, and patients most likely will continue to self-treat while consulting with biomedical health care providers. Thus, rather than ignoring the fact that your patient is self-treating, assess the patient's use of self-care and then consider negotiating a compromise.

Example: A chronically ill 78-year-old man with osteoarthritis was being examined by a nurse at an ambulatory care clinic. While taking his vital signs, the nurse asked the patient why the skin on his wrist was broken and irritated. The patient explained that he had been wearing a copper bracelet for his arthritis. He hoped that the bracelet might work, but thus far it had only made his skin sore.

The nurse smiled. "I know of other patients who have tried these bracelets. Have you done anything else for your arthritis?" The patient replied, "My pain has been so bad that I sprayed my elbow and knee with some lubricant I bought at the drugstore. But it hasn't helped much." The nurse again asked the patient if he had done anything more for the arthritis. The patient said that a friend had returned from Mexico with some pills that were supposed to reduce joint swelling, but they were not working either.

Note that by using a nonjudgmental approach and by exploring the patient's answers in depth, the nurse was able to learn a great deal about the patient's methods of self-care. Using this information, the nurse developed the following nursing diagnoses:

- Impaired skin integrity related to pressure from copper bracelet

- Risk for infection related to broken skin

- Chronic pain related to chronic disability

Next, the nurse, in an attempt to negotiate with the patient, asked, "Are you planning to continue self-treating your joint swelling? If you are, are you also willing to take the medication as prescribed?" If the patient does decide to use both self-care and biomedical therapies, he may attribute any improvement to his natural remedies.

ELICITING INFORMATION FROM THE PATIENT'S FAMILY AND SUPPORT GROUP

When approached with concern and respect, the patient's family can provide you and the physician with vital information. Consider members of the patient's family as cultural informants and allies in providing care. The first steps in working with the family are to (1) survey family members and (2) identify a family liaison.

Surveying the family involves identifying family members and clarifying their relationship to the patient. It is important to learn about members of the patient's immediate social support network, the patient's extended support network, and the patient's family history. Surveying is particularly helpful when caring for families in cultural transition (e.g., immigrant families and recently arrived refugees).

In some situations, you may want to develop a **genogram**, which is a tool for recording and visualizing family information. Figure 11-2 provides an example of a genogram. Note that the genogram displays the causes of death among family members and the age at which each deceased family member died.

•••• COMMUNICATION CONSIDERATIONS ••••

Assure family members that you want to learn about the patient's family in order to understand the patient's position and role within the family.

Once you become acquainted with the patient's family, choose one member to act as a *liaison* to the entire family, both immediate and extended. You will probably select the family member who is the most acculturated to mainstream American values. You can inform the **family liaison** about the patient's condition and ask the liaison to tell other family members. You can also ask that the liaison communicate the ideas and feelings of family members back to you.

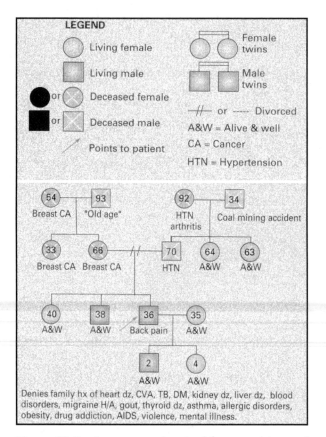

Figure 11-2 A genogram is a tool for organizing and visualizing family information.

To learn about the patient's illness from the family's perspective, ask a family member (or the family liaison) the following questions:

• How long have your family members been in this country?

• What are family members doing to help the patient deal with pain or other symptoms?

• How has the patient's illness affected family relationships? *Note:* In extended families, the patient's illness may have disrupted that person's role (or roles) in the family as primary breadwinner, primary caregiver, or counselor, for example.

• How has the patient's illness affected family income? Is the patient the primary wage earner?

Example: A Cambodian man in his early twenties was hospitalized after being hit by a car. The nurse learned that the man had two younger sisters who were attending school, and his elderly father was in poor health. The patient was emotionally devastated because he was the primary wage earner in his family. He worried that his family would suffer severe socioeconomic stress because he was now hospitalized.

- Do relatives want to be involved in every aspect of decision making that concerns the patient?

For instance, in many Hispanic families, the adult children will support each others' decisions regarding care for an aging parent. The son or daughter may request that the nurse speak with family members first, to protect the patient from having to make numerous decisions. This attitude is in contrast to many elderly Greek, East Indian, and Iranian patients, who prefer not to discuss any health issues in the presence of their children.

In most cases, family members will be glad to talk to you about their loved one's illness. However, some relatives—especially immigrant families and refugees who have recently moved to the United States from a totalitarian country—may be suspicious of an authority figure who asks too many questions. You will need to first gain the trust of families who have experienced life as refugees before they will be willing to share personal information with you.

REFERENCES

Bailey, E. J. (1991). *Urban African American health care.* Indianapolis: University Press of America.

Benner, P. (1984). *From novice to expert.* Menlo Park, CA: Addison-Wesley.

Buchwald, D., Caralis, P. V., & Gany, F. (1994). Caring for patients in a multicultural society. *Patient Care, 28*(11), 105–123.

Bushy, A. (1992). Cultural considerations for primary health care: Where do self-care and folk medicine fit? *Holistic Nurse Practitioner, 6*(3), 10–18.

Campinha-Bacote, J. (1995). The quest for cultural competence in nursing care. *Nursing Forum, 30*(4), 19–25.

Chester, B., & Holtan, N. (1992). Working with refugee survivors of torture. (Cross-Cultural Medicine—A Decade Later). *Western Journal of Medicine, 157*, 301–304.

Dreyfus, S., & Dreyfus, H. (1980). A five-stage model of the mental activities involved in directed skill acquisition. Unpublished report. University of California at Berkeley.

Evans, C. A., & Cunningham, B. A. (1996). Caring for the ethnic elder. *Geriatric Nursing*, *17*(3), 105–110.

Fong, C. M. (1985). Ethnicity and nursing practice. *Topics in Clinical Nursing*, *7*(3), 1–10.

Germain, C. P. (1992). Cultural care: A bridge between sickness, illness, and disease. *Holistic Nurse Practitioner*, *6*(3), 1–9.

Jackson, L. E. (1993). Understanding, eliciting, and negotiating clients' multicultural health beliefs. *Nurse Practitioner*, *18*(4), 30–34.

Jezewski, M. A. (1990). Culture brokering in migrant farmworkers care. *Western Journal of Nursing Research*, *12*(4), 497–513.

Leininger, M. (1978). *Transcultural nursing: Theories, concepts, and practices.* New York: Wiley.

Levin, S. J., Like, R. C., & Gottlieb, J. E. (2000). ETHIC: A framework for culturally competent clinical practice. *Patient Care*, *34*(9), 188–189.

Mauksch, L. B., & Roesler, T. (1990). Expanding the context of the patient's explanatory model using circular questioning. *Family Systems Medicine*, *8*(1), 3–13.

Rosenbaun, J. N. (1991). A cultural assessment guide: Learning cultural sensitivity. *The Canadian Nurse*, *87*(4), 32–33.

Terrance, O. (1994). *Comprehensive accreditation manual for hospitals 1995.* Joint Commission on Accreditation of Healthcare Organizations.

SUGGESTED READINGS

Andrews, M. M., & Boyle, J. S. (2003). *Transcultural concepts in nursing care* (4th ed.). Philadelphia: Lippincott.

Bonder, B., & Martin, L. (2001). Achieving cultural competence: The challenge for clients and health care workers in a multicultural society. *Generations*, *25*(1), 35.

Charnes, L. S. (1992). Meeting patients' spiritual needs: The Jewish perspective. *Holistic Nurse Practitioner*, *6*(3), 64–72.

Gardenswartz, L., & Rowe, A. (1998). *Improving communications in a diverse environment: Managing diversity in health care.* San Francisco: Jossey-Bass.

Giger, J. N., & Davidhizar, R. E. (1999). *Transcultural nursing: Assessment and intervention* (3rd ed.). St. Louis: Mosby.

Jandt, F. E. (2003). *An introduction to intercultural communication: Identities in a global community.* Thousand Oaks, CA: Sage

Lipson, J., & Dibble S. (1996). *Culture and nursing care: A pocket guide.* San Francisco: UCSF Nursing Press.

Martin, J., Nakayama, T., & Flores, L. (2002). *Readings in intercultural communications: Experiences & contexts.* Boston: McGraw-Hill.

Muñoz, C. (2001). Addressing the linguistic and cultural needs of case management clients. *Case Manager, 12*(6), 58–63.

Narayan, M. C. (1997). Cultural assessment in home health care. *Home Health Care Nurse, 15*(10), 663–670.

Porter, C. P., & Villarruel, A. M. (1993). Nursing research with African American and Hispanic people: Guidelines for action. *Nursing Outlook, 41*(2), 59–67.

Purnell, L. D., & Paulanka, B. J. (2003). *Transcultural health care: A culturally competent approach* (2nd ed.). Philadelphia: Davis.

Samovar, L. A., & Porter, R. E. (2003). *Intercultural communication: A reader.* Belmont, CA: Wadsworth.

Spector, R. E. (2000). *A guide to heritage assessment and health traditions.* Upper Saddle River, NJ: Prentice Hall.

Stewart, M. (1998). Nurses need to strengthen cultural competence for next century to ensure quality patient care. *American Nurse, 30*(1), 26–27.

Wenger, A. F. Z. (1993). Cultural meaning of symptoms. *Holistic Nurse Practitioner, 7*(2), 22–35.

CHAPTER 12

Developing Culturally Appropriate Nursing Diagnoses

KEY TERMS

- Defining Characteristics
- Diagnostic Label
- Disturbed Thought Processes
- Etiology
- External Locus of Control
- Impaired Social Interaction
- Impaired Verbal Communication
- Internal Locus of Control
- Knowledge Deficient
- Noncompliance
- North American Nursing Diagnosis Association (NANDA)
- Nursing Diagnosis Taxonomy
- Powerlessness

OBJECTIVES

After completing this chapter, you should be able to:

- Define *nursing diagnosis* and describe the three parts of a nursing diagnosis.
- Discuss the six transcultural concerns regarding NANDA's nursing diagnosis taxonomy that were voiced by Madeline Leininger.
- List and discuss six nursing diagnoses that can potentially hinder transcultural communication.

- State how a culturally sensitive patient assessment, free of bias and unfounded assumptions, leads directly to the formulation of culturally appropriate nursing diagnoses.

- Discuss the role of validation and evaluation in the development of culturally appropriate nursing diagnoses.

- Identify at least four techniques nurses can use to communicate and implement appropriate nursing diagnoses.

INTRODUCTION

For over a century, nurses have tried to define themselves. As nurses, we are constantly in pursuit of the perfect definition, the perfect set of criteria for practice, the perfect solution to the *what is nursing* question. Our attempts to define and identify our place at the health care table have been many and varied. Within the last quarter century, nurses have tried to define and classify nursing by developing and using a **nursing diagnosis taxonomy**. This taxonomy was spearheaded and promoted by the **North American Nursing Diagnosis Association (NANDA)**, an organization that was founded in the 1980s.

NANDA defines a nursing diagnosis as: "A clinical judgment about individual, family, or community responses to actual and potential health problems/life processes." According to NANDA, "Nursing diagnoses provide the basis for selection of nursing interventions to achieve outcomes for which the nurse is accountable" (NANDA, 2003). Nursing diagnoses are ideally based on thorough, individualized patient assessments. Once assessment data have been gathered, the next step is to identify cues or patterns that may indicate a problem, a risk for a problem, or a health-promoting behavior that the nurse needs to support and enhance.

A nursing diagnosis has three parts:

1. The **diagnostic label** or problem statement: for example, *impaired skin integrity*.

2. The **etiology** or reason for that label or problem: for example, *impaired skin integrity related to immobility*.

3. A list of **defining characteristics** that validate the diagnosis: for example, reddened skin areas at bony prominences, reported discomfort at bony prominences, bed rest status, and loss of ability to move or walk are defining characteristics of *impaired skin integrity related to immobility*.

To organize individual nursing diagnoses into a taxonomy, nursing theorists grouped nursing diagnoses into the following nine human response patterns (Bolander, 1994):

1. Exchanging
2. Communicating
3. Relating
4. Valuing
5. Choosing
6. Moving
7. Perceiving
8. Knowing
9. Feeling

This method of organization allowed NANDA representatives to create an underlying structure, or taxonomy, of multidimensional sets of labels, ranging from concrete, observable, and clearly measurable labels (e.g., *total incontinence*) to abstract labels, which are more theoretical and less clinically useful (e.g., *personal identity disturbance*). Selected NANDA-approved nursing diagnoses by human response patterns are listed on pages 226–228.

Even though thousands of nurses are committed to using nursing diagnoses, and the NANDA list continues to grow, the nursing diagnosis movement is not without controversy. One major controversy revolves around those nursing diagnoses that are sometimes used in culturally biased and inappropriate ways.

For example, the nursing diagnosis of *noncompliance* can have judgmental overtones when applied to patients from diverse cultures. Patients from non-Western cultures who want to follow their own traditional methods of healing instead of Western medical practices are sometimes unfairly labeled as *noncompliant*. A better nursing diagnosis for these patients might be *Different Cultural Values* or *Different Cultural Beliefs*. Thus, transcultural nursing specialists need to improve the wording of nursing diagnoses to make them more culturally sensitive and appropriate (Ward-Collins, 1998).

This chapter will discuss: (1) how nursing diagnoses can potentially hinder transcultural communication and cultural competence in nursing and (2) how to formulate and communicate nursing diagnoses that are culturally appropriate. We will also present six nursing diagnoses that may be culturally biased, and we will describe ways to make such diagnoses more helpful.

SELECTED NANDA-APPROVED NURSING DIAGNOSES BY HUMAN RESPONSE PATTERNS

PATTERN 1: EXCHANGING

Imbalanced Nutrition: More Than Body Requirements

Imbalanced Nutrition: Less Than Body Requirements

Imbalanced Nutrition: Risk for More Than Body Requirements

Infection, Risk for

Body Temperature, Risk for Imbalanced

Hypothermia

Hyperthermia

Thermoregulation, Ineffective

Dysreflexia, Autonomic, Risk for

Constipation

Perceived Constipation

Risk for Constipation

Diarrhea

Bowel Incontinence

Urinary Elimination: Impaired or Readiness

Stress, Urinary

Reflex, Urinary

Urge, Urinary

Functional, Urinary

Total, Urinary

Retention, Urinary

Tissue Perfusion: Ineffective (Renal, cerebral, cardiopulmonary, gastrointestinal, peripheral)

Fluid Volume Excess

Fluid Volume Deficit

Risk for Fluid Volume Deficit

Cardiac Output

Gas Exchange

Airway Clearance

Breathing Pattern

Sustain Ventilation

Ventilatory Weaning Response, Dysfunctional

Injury, Risk for

Suffocation, Risk for

Poisoning, Risk for

Trauma, Risk for

Aspiration, Risk for

Disuse Syndrome, Risk for

Protection: Ineffective

Tissue Integrity: Impaired

Oral Mucous Membrane: Impaired

Skin Integrity: Impaired

Risk for Impaired Skin Integrity

Adaptive Capacity: Decreased Intracranial

Energy Field: Disturbed

PATTERN 2: COMMUNICATING

Verbal Communication: Impaired

PATTERN 3: RELATING

Social Interaction: Impaired

Social Isolation

Loneliness: Impaired

Role Performance: Ineffective

Impaired Parenting

Risk for Impaired Parenting

Sexual Dysfunction

Family Processes

Caregiver Role Strain

Risk for Caregiver Role Strain

Family Process: Interrupted

Family Process: Readiness for Enhanced

Family Process: Dysfunctional Alcoholism

Parental Role Conflict

Sexuality Pattern: Ineffective

PATTERN 4: VALUING

Spiritual Distress (distress of the human spirit)

Potential for Enhanced Spiritual Well-Being

PATTERN 5: CHOOSING

Ineffective Coping

Impaired Adjustment

Defensive Coping

Denial: Ineffective

Ineffective Family Coping: Disabled

Family Coping: Compromised

Family Coping: Readiness for Enhanced

Readiness for Enhanced Community Coping

Ineffective Community Coping

Ineffective Management of Therapeutic Regimen (Individuals)

Noncompliance (Specify)

Therapeutic Regimen Management: Effective

Therapeutic Regimen Management: Ineffective

Therapeutic Regimen Management: Ineffective, Community

Decisional Conflict (Specify)

Health Seeking, Behaviors (Specify)

PATTERN 6: MOVING

Impaired Physical Mobility

Risk for Peripheral Neurovascular Dysfunction

Risk for Perioperative Positioning Injury

Activity Intolerance

Fatigue

Risk for Activity Intolerance

Sleep Pattern: Disturbed

Diversional Activity: Deficient

Home Maintenance, Impaired

Ineffective Health Maintenance

Feeding Self-Care Deficit

Impaired Swallowing

Ineffective Breast-feeding

Interrupted Breast-feeding

Effective Breast-feeding

Ineffective Infant Feeding Pattern

Bathing/Hygiene Self-Care Deficit

Dressing/Grooming Self-Care Deficit

Toileting Self-Care Deficit

Risk for Disproportionate Growth and Development

Relocation Stess Syndrome

Risk for Disorganized Infant Behavior

Disorganized Infant Behavior

Readiness for Enhanced Organized Infant Behavior

PATTERN 7: PERCEIVING

Disturbed Body Image

Self-Esteem, Risk for Situational: Low

Chronic Low Self-Esteem

Situational Low Self-Esteem

Self-Esteem, Chronic Low

Self-Esteem, Situational Low

Disturbed Personal Identity Disturbance

(continues)

Sensory/Perceptual Alterations
(Specify) (Visual, Auditory,
Kinesthetic, Gustatory, Tactile,
Olfactory)
Unilateral Neglect
Hopelessness
Powerlessness

PATTERN 8: KNOWING
Knowledge Deficit (Specify)
Impaired Environmental
Interpretation Syndrome
Acute Confusion
Chronic Confusion
Disturbed Thought Processes
Impaired Memory

PATTERN 9: FEELING
Acute Pain
Chronic Pain
Dysfunctional Grieving
Anticipatory Grieving
Risk for Violence: Self-Directed or
Other-Directed
Risk for Self-Mutilation
Post-Trauma Syndrome
Rape-Trauma Syndrome
Rape-Trauma Syndrome: Compound
Reaction
Rape-Trauma Syndrome: Silent
Reaction
Anxiety
Fear

NEW, DELETED, AND REVISED NURSING DIAGNOSES DEFINITIONS & CLASSIFICATION (2003–2004)

NEW
PATTERN 1: EXCHANGING
Readiness for Enhanced Communication
Readiness for Enhanced Coping
Readiness for Enhanced Family Process
Readiness for Enhanced Fluid Balance
Readiness for Enhanced Knowledge
(Specify)
Readiness for Enhanced Nutrition
Readiness for Enhanced Parenting
Readiness for Enhanced Sleep
Readiness for Enhanced Self-Concept
Readiness for Enhanced Management
of Therapeutic Regimen
Readiness for Enhanced Urinary
Elimination

DELETED
PATTERN 1: EXCHANGING
Colonic Constipation

REVISED
PATTERN 1: EXCHANGING
Nausea
Readiness for Enhanced Spiritual
Well-Being
Spiritual Distress

PATTERN 2: COMMUNICATING
Impaired Verbal Communication

PATTERN 5: CHOOSING
Ineffective Community Coping
Noncompliance (Specify)

Reprinted with permission of the North American Nursing Diagnosis Association. (2003). NANDA Nursing
Diagnoses: Definitions and Classification, 2003–2004. Philadelphia: Author.

CULTURAL BIASES IN NURSING DIAGNOSES THAT HINDER COMMUNICATION

Although the nursing diagnoses developed by NANDA have been successfully applied to patients from the American mainstream culture, they have sometimes obscured and distorted the problems of patients from diverse cultures. With this problem in mind, Leininger (1990) identified the following six transcultural concerns regarding NANDA's nursing diagnosis taxonomy:

1. The current nursing diagnosis taxonomy is based on Anglo-American Western cultural standards and values and has limited relevance to other cultures or countries.

2. NANDA language prevents non-Anglicized nurses from communicating and contributing beliefs and values from their own unique cultures.

3. NANDA diagnostic categories seem ethnocentric.

4. NANDA categories focus on negative conditions and are medically oriented.

5. NANDA category norms do not seem to consider transcultural variations.

6. NANDA diagnoses, when used around the world, present ethical issues.

Given these problems, Leininger concluded that the NANDA diagnostic classification system needs to be reevaluated, refocused, and reworded in order to be transculturally useful and meaningful. One important step is to build a new or revised *taxonomy* of diagnostic labels that will acknowledge that patients have different cultural backgrounds, which, in turn, affect their beliefs concerning health and illness. Also, NANDA's defining characteristics need to be more specific for different cultures (Lunney, 1994).

NURSING DIAGNOSES THAT MAY BE CULTURALLY BIASED

All nursing diagnoses, when applied incorrectly, have the potential of being more harmful than helpful. There are six nursing diagnoses that can be especially troublesome when the patient is from another cultural heritage. These diagnoses are

1. Verbal Communication: Impaired

2. Noncompliance

3. Social Interaction: Impaired

4. Disturbed Thought Processes

5. Knowledge Deficient

6. Powerlessness

Three Revised Nursing Diagnoses

To help remedy the problem of culturally insensitive nursing diagnoses, Geissler (1991) surveyed 254 transcultural nursing experts from the United States and seven other countries. On the basis of the survey results, Geissler rewrote the NANDA definitions and defining characteristics for the following three problematic diagnoses: impaired verbal communication, noncompliance, and impaired social interaction (Geissler, 1991).

Impaired Verbal Communication. NANDA defines **impaired verbal communication** as "the state in which an individual experiences a decreased or absent ability to use or to understand language in human interaction." Geissler's study reevaluated this NANDA definition from a transcultural perspective. The study concluded that neither the nurse nor the patient has impaired verbal communication when both are able to speak and comprehend their own language. Thus, it is incorrect to use the diagnosis of impaired verbal communication for patients who do not speak English.

Another major concern over NANDA's current use and definition of impaired verbal communication is that it eliminates the enormous amount of communication that takes place at the *nonverbal* level. Nonverbal communications are strongly influenced by cultural differences in values, beliefs, and customs, as well as differences in the meaning of gestures, facial expressions, eye contact, use of personal and interpersonal space, touch, and posture. Therefore, etiologies for this diagnostic label should be identified as cultural differences in language or in the *expression* of that language or both (Geissler, 1991).

Because the NANDA definition for this diagnosis ignores language differences, study participants reworded and redefined impaired verbal communication as "the state in which an individual is unable to speak/ understand the dominant language of the health care delivery system when the barrier is not secondary to physical or psychological disorders" (Geissler, 1991).

Example: A culturally appropriate nursing diagnosis that takes both verbal and nonverbal communication into account: "Altered verbal communication related to differences in language and cultural expression." These are the defining characteristics for *impaired verbal communication* that met NANDA criteria and were also acceptable to the study participants:

- Unable to speak dominant language.
- Speaks or verbalizes with difficulty.
- Difficulty expressing thought verbally.

Noncompliance. NANDA defines **noncompliance** as "a person's informed decision not to adhere to a therapeutic recommendation." Because each culture has its own methods for maintaining health and avoiding illness, this definition is both limited and biased. NANDA's definition does not take into account the many *cultural reasons* patients decide not to adhere to a therapeutic recommendation.

For instance, patients may not agree with the nurse's identification of the cause or causes for the problem. Also, patients with different cultural beliefs may not value the same outcomes, treatments, and interventions as the nurse.

Biological variations may also affect a patient's compliance with treatment. Race affects therapeutic ranges and thresholds of medications, treatment efficacy, and occurrences of disorders that may develop as a result of treatment (iatrogenic disorders). For example, people from different races may metabolize and respond differently to medications, and they may experience different side effects and toxic effects.

Besides biological variations, there are many other possible reasons for nonadherence to prescribed medical treatment. For example, patients may not have access to *transportation*, thus they cannot make and meet appointments. Patients may not have the *financial resources* to purchase medications or medical equipment such as dressings or syringes. Patients may have a culturally linked *time orientation* that includes only the present. As a response to a plan of therapy, these patients might say: "If I am feeling well right now, why do I need to take my insulin or blood pressure pills?"

In practice, the term *noncompliance* is more an attitude than a nursing diagnosis. The notion of noncompliance is based on a Western medical model heritage that reinforces the idea that the health care provider always knows best. Just because a patient exercises the right not to follow a provider's recommendations does not warrant this negative, even elitist, label. With this thought in mind, the 245 nurses who participated in Geissler's study recommended changing this diagnostic label from *noncompliance* to *nonadherence*. Their definition for *nonadherence* reads, "A value conflict in which a person uses own rules of compliance (adherence) which differ from the dominant culture" (Geissler, 1991).

> **Example:** A culturally appropriate nursing diagnosis: "Nonadherence to clinic appointment schedule related to inability to access public or private transportation." These are the defining characteristics for *noncompliance* that met NANDA criteria and were also acceptable to the transcultural nurses in Geissler's study:
>
> - Behavior indicative of failure to adhere.
> - Failure to keep appointments.

Impaired Social Interaction. NANDA defines **impaired social interaction** as "The state in which an individual participates in an insufficient or excessive quantity or ineffective quality of social exchange." Geissler (1991) writes:

> This definition fails to consider in what setting the problem exists: within the dominant culture, the patient's own culture, or both. The reasons for the patient's interaction difficulties must also be identified.

Geissler's study group revised this definition to read: "The state in which an individual is observed to have or verbally expresses conflict in social exchange with members of the dominant culture or with members of own cultural group" (Geissler, 1991). Actually, the experts had difficulty with the word *impaired* and preferred *altered social interaction* because of its cultural implications and context.

COMMUNICATION CONSIDERATIONS

It is important to recognize that social behavior that may appear to be impaired or altered within one cultural situation may be perfectly normal and even condoned within another cultural setting. Thus, from the patient's standpoint, impaired social interaction could really be the nurse's problem.

A thorough cultural assessment is the key to understanding social interactive behavior. Because a patient's culture, family background, and social behavior are enmeshed, it is important to survey the patient's support system, including family members and close friends. When possible, it may help to observe patient–family social interaction. It is also vital to learn about the accessibility of family members and whether they will be able to help the patient after discharge (see Chapter 10).

For example, most patients have family members with them when they arrive at the health care facility, and most return to their family and homes upon discharge. Unfortunately, patients from other countries may not have family or close friends in the United States, and they may arrive at and leave the hospital alone. In these cases, you will need to anticipate the problems that may arise for the patient as a result of altered social interactions.

Example: A culturally appropriate nursing diagnosis for patients with this problem might read: "Altered social interactions related to international distance between patient and perceived and valued social support system." These are the defining characteristics for *impaired (altered) social interaction* that met NANDA criteria and were also acceptable to the study participants:

- Verbalized or observed discomfort in social situations.

- Verbalized or observed inability to receive or communicate a satisfying sense of belonging, caring, interest, or shared history.

Other Nursing Diagnoses

There are other nursing diagnoses that nurses sometimes use in a culturally inappropriate way and that need to be revised to reflect patients' cultural differences. These diagnoses include altered thought processes, knowledge deficit, and powerlessness. See additional diagnoses on page 229.

Disturbed Thought Processes. NANDA defines **disturbed thought processes** as "A state in which a person experiences a disruption in cognitive operations and activities." This ethnocentric definition does not take cultural differences into account, thus creating a nursing diagnosis that can be inaccurate and potentially damaging to the patient.

For instance, nurses from Western cultures sometimes misdiagnose culture-specific thought processes and behavior as being pathologic. A nurse might misdiagnose a patient from another culture as having *disturbed thought processes* if the nurse witnessed the patient walking backwards into a room, sleeping on the floor completely encased in sheets and blankets, holding tightly to icons that appear valueless, speaking about spells or voodoo, or rubbing coins on the skin, causing lesions and bruising. This diagnosis as worded might be incorrect because the patient's thinking, although not in sync with Western thought, may be perfectly in tune with the patient's cultural beliefs and values. Thus, the definition of this diagnosis needs to be reworded to reflect cultural differences in thought patterns.

Knowledge Deficient. NANDA defines **knowledge deficient** as "absence or deficiency of cognitive information related to specific topic." Knowledge deficient is often incorrectly used as the diagnostic label or problem statement of a nursing diagnosis; for example, "Knowledge deficient related to measures to prevent constipation." It is better to use knowledge deficient as the *etiology* or reason for the problem; for instance, "High risk for constipation related to knowledge deficient of high-fiber foods and adequate fluid intake."

A diagnosis of knowledge deficient can be applied to the nurse as well as to the patient. Remember that patients may be very knowledgeable about their own health care needs but unable to express this information in English without an interpreter. Patients may also know a great deal about the complementary (alternative) healing methods used in their culture but know little about Western therapies. Conversely, you may be very knowledgeable about nursing and biomedical therapies but have a knowledge deficient in regard to the patient's culture and its methods for treating disease.

● • • • **COMMUNICATION CONSIDERATIONS** • • • ●

Do not assume that patients from other cultures lack knowledge just because they are unfamiliar with biomedical practices and Western culture. If you acknowledge and respect what the patient knows, the patient is much more likely to acknowledge and respect what you know.

Powerlessness. NANDA defines **powerlessness** as the "perception that one's own action will not significantly affect an outcome; a perceived lack of control over a current situation or immediate happening." This definition does not take a patient's cultural background and beliefs into account. According to the Western medical model, all patients should make their own decisions, value personal responsibility and autonomy, and seek all health-related information from the medical community. However, some cultures may not promote patient autonomy. In some cultures, it is customary for family members or a cultural or religious leader to make decisions on behalf of the patient. Within these cultures, patients may not perceive themselves as powerless or lacking control, because it is customary for family to take control during a time of illness.

Moreover, a person's *locus of control* determines the extent to which an individual feels more powerful or more powerless. *Locus of control* refers to the degree of control people feel that they have over events in their lives. Patients with an **internal locus of control** feel that they have some control over events; this is a common belief among middle-class Americans. For example, when diagnosed with mild hypertension, these patients believe that they can take control of their health by setting up a plan of exercise, losing weight, avoiding salty foods, and reducing stress.

Patients with an **external locus of control** believe that they have little control over life events. For example, some Mexicans, Appalachians, and South Americans feel that they cannot control what happens to them. When diagnosed with hypertension, these patients might not try to change their lifestyle because they feel that what they do makes little difference. These individuals may believe that fate, luck, and chance, not their own actions, control their health (see Chapter 15).

It is easy to assume that *all* patients from certain cultures have an external locus of control. Using such stereotypical thinking, some nurses might diagnose and treat these patients as if they are powerless. This is a serious misdiagnosis. First of all, patients should never be stereotyped according to culture because patients are first and foremost individuals. Also, patients may have a locus of control that is completely opposite to that which is valued in their culture.

When your patients do feel powerless, it is important to find ways to empower them and help them feel more in control. For example, Herman (1994) studied a group of Hispanic women who thought of themselves as powerless and who behaved in accordance with NANDA's definition of powerlessness. However, when a health professional acted as an advocate on their behalf, these women started to perceive themselves as more powerful and as having some control over their environment and their health.

WRITING CULTURALLY APPROPRIATE NURSING DIAGNOSES

Because nursing diagnoses are clinical judgments about a patient's responses to health and illness, they provide a foundation for culturally competent care. The first step in developing culturally appropriate nursing diagnoses is to perform an *accurate and thorough cultural assessment* of the patient. It is important to identify the patient's cultural heritage, history, values, beliefs, and preferences without stereotyping the patient (see Chapter 11).

COMMUNICATION CONSIDERATIONS

To assume that all nursing diagnoses can be indiscriminately applied to all patients impairs quality nurse–patient relationships. Remember to write individualized nursing diagnoses for each patient, regardless of that person's cultural background.

As you do your assessment, keep in mind that the degree to which people adhere to cultural beliefs and practices is related to their level of *acculturation*. People who have recently entered the United States often were educated outside of American borders, live in close ethnic communities, prefer their native language, continue to travel to and from their country of origin, and routinely interact with community elders. As a result, these individuals may be less acculturated and have different health beliefs and practices than those who have chosen to adopt American behaviors and language (Pachter, 1994). In these cases, take special care that you use nursing diagnoses in a culturally sensitive manner.

COMMUNICATION CONSIDERATIONS

Before you compile your problem list and make your diagnosis, remember to elicit the patient's explanation (explanatory model) for why an illness developed (see Chapter 11). Encourage patients to discuss their viewpoints about health and illness, and incorporate these data into the etiology or reason section of your nursing diagnosis. For example, "Nonadherence to prescribed diet related to dietary practices valued within the culture."

Before implementing nursing diagnoses, *validate* your diagnoses with your patients and their families. Validating is particularly important when patients are from another culture. For example, you might diagnose a patient as suffering from impaired social interaction when the person is a newcomer to the United States and without family or friends in this country.

Even sound nursing diagnoses need to be continually *evaluated and updated* as the patient's health status changes and as the person learns to cope with problems. For example, you might initially diagnose a Hispanic patient who seems passive as suffering from powerlessness. However, once the patient feels empowered by having a strong advocate, that diagnosis becomes irrelevant.

····· COMMUNICATION CONSIDERATIONS ·····

How we formulate nursing diagnoses can positively or negatively affect patient care. Nursing diagnoses and patient care need to be flexible, supportive, intelligent, and most of all, sensitive to cultural differences.

PROMOTING CULTURALLY APPROPRIATE DIAGNOSES

Nurses can communicate and implement appropriate nursing diagnoses by conferring with peers, other health care professionals, and transcultural nursing specialists. This communication may take place at the individual, group, and professional levels. Specific ways in which nurses can help promote more culturally appropriate nursing diagnoses are to:

- Participate in care conferences, team meetings, and shift reports.
- Join and participate in clinical care committees.
- Individualize and revise standardized care plans and critical pathways within nursing units and health care facilities.
- Join professional nursing organizations and work on projects related to culturally competent nursing care and appropriate nursing diagnoses.
- Participate in nursing research.
- Write about clinical applications of nursing diagnoses for the professional nursing press. This documentation could be as simple as a letter to the editor or as involved as a manuscript.
- Help professional peers understand the cultural differences of patients they care for by hosting workshops or training sessions, speaking at conferences, and creating networks.
- Collaborate with other professionals (such as radiologists, physicians, social workers, respiratory specialists) to create an accessible, flexible, culturally sensitive health care environment for each patient and community.
- Collaborate with folk healers or culturally sanctioned healers and share ideas, experiences, and discoveries with them. You might invite these healers to class, clinical, or organization meetings and ask them to discuss and demonstrate their healing methods.

- Use NANDA's request for participation by all nurses as a vehicle for influencing our current and future professional nursing diagnosis endeavors.

- Identify culturally sensitive defining characteristics for existing nursing diagnostic labels and report these to NANDA and other interested organizations such as the Transcultural Nursing Society.

COMMUNICATION CONSIDERATIONS

Nurses who understand the importance of transcultural communication can and should participate in the process of formulating, refining, and implementing culturally sensitive diagnoses. The active participation of nurses in formulating nursing diagnoses will improve the lives and health of our culturally diverse patients.

REFERENCES

Bolander, V. R. (1994). *Sorensen and Luckmann's basic nursing: A psychophysiologic approach* (3rd ed.). Philadelphia: Saunders.

Geissler, E. M. (1991). Nursing diagnoses of culturally diverse patients. *International Nursing Review, 38*(5), 150–152.

Herman, M. (1994). Integrating culture diversity into present nursing diagnosis taxonomy. In R. M. Carroll-Johnson & M. Paquette (Eds.), *Classification of nursing diagnoses: Proceedings of the tenth conference* (p. 385). Philadelphia: Lippincott.

Leininger, M. (1990). Issues, questions, and concerns related to the nursing diagnosis cultural movement from a transcultural nursing perspective. *Journal of Transcultural Nursing, 2*(1), 23–32.

Lunney, M. (1994). Nursing diagnosis in cross cultural settings: Commentary. *Nursing Diagnosis, 5*(4), 172–173.

North American Nursing Diagnosis Association (NANDA). (2003). *Nursing diagnoses: Definitions and classification, 2003–2004.* Philadelphia: Author.

Pachter, L. M. (1994). Culture and clinical care: Folk illness beliefs and behaviors and their implications for health care delivery. *Journal of the American Medical Association, 271*(9), 690–694.

Ward-Collins, D. (1998). "Noncompliant": Isn't there a better way to say it? *American Journal of Nursing, 98*(5), 27–32.

SUGGESTED READINGS

AAN Expert Panel on Culturally Competent Health Care. (1992). *Nursing Outlook, 40*(6), 277–283.

Andrews, M. M., & Boyle, J. S. (2003). *Transcultural concepts in nursing care* (4th ed.). Philadelphia: Lippincott.

Blackhall, L. J., Murphy, S. T., Frank, G., Michel, V., & Azen, S. (1995). Ethnicity and attitudes toward patient autonomy. *Journal of the American Medical Association, 274*(10), 820–825.

Campinha-Bacote, J. (1994). Transcultural psychiatric nursing: Diagnostic and treatment issues. *Journal of Psychosocial Nursing and Mental Health Services, 32*(8), 41–46.

Campinha-Bacote, J., & Muñoz, C. (2001). A guiding framework for delivering culturally competent services in case management. *Case Manager, 12*(2), 48–52.

Capers, C. F. (1994). Mental health issues and African-Americans. *Nursing Clinics of North America, 29*(1), 57–64.

Doenges, M. E., & Moorhouse, M. F. (2002). *Nurse's pocket guide: Nursing diagnoses with interventions* (5th ed.). Philadelphia: Davis.

Geissler, E. M. (1992). Nursing diagnoses: A study of cultural relevance. *Journal of Professional Nursing, 8*(5), 301–307.

Giger, J. N., & Davidhizar, R. E. (2003). *Transcultural nursing: Assessment and intervention* (4th ed.). St. Louis: Mosby.

Heliker, D. (1992). Reevaluation of a nursing diagnosis: Spiritual distress. *Nursing Forum, 27*(4), 15–20.

Kritek, P. B. (1986). Diagnostics: The struggle to classify our diagnoses. *American Journal of Nursing, 86*(6), 722–723.

Lester, N. (1998). Cultural competence: A nursing dialogue. *American Journal of Nursing, 90*(8), 26–34.

Lester, N. (1998). Cultural competence: A nursing dialogue (Part II). *American Journal of Nursing, 90*(9), 36–44.

Meleis, A. I. (1997). *Theoretical nursing: Development and progress* (3rd ed.). Philadelphia: Lippincott.

National Alliance for Hispanic Health. (2000). *A primer for cultural proficiency: Towards quality health services for Hispanics.* Washington, DC: Estrella Press.

North American Nursing Diagnosis Association (NANDA). (1996). *Nursing diagnoses: Definitions and classification, 1997-1998.* Philadelphia: NANDA.

North American Nursing Diagnosis Association (NANDA). (1999). *New, deleted, and revised nursing diagnoses: Definitions and classification, 1999–2000.* Philadelphia: NANDA.

Reardon-Anderson, J., Capps, R., & Fix, M. (2002). *The health and well-being of children in immigrant families* (Series B, p. B–52). Washington, DC: The Urban Institute.

Spector, R. E. (2004). *Cultural diversity in health and illness* (6th ed.). Upper Saddle River, NJ: Prentice Hall.

Wieck, K. L. (1996). Diagnostic language consistency among multicultural English-speaking nurses. *Nursing Diagnosis, 7*(2), 70–78.

Wuest, J. (1993). Removing the shackles: A feminist critique of noncompliance. *Nursing Outlook, 41,* 217–224.

UNIT THREE
EVALUATION

EVALUATING YOUR ABILITY TO ELICIT ASSESSMENT DATA AND DEVELOP NURSING DIAGNOSES

The following exercises will highlight some of the concepts that were discussed in this unit. They will also help you identify and evaluate the progress that you have made in your ability to culturally assess patients and identify and use culturally appropriate nursing diagnoses.

Exercise One: Evaluating Your Personal Objectives

Before you began studying this unit, you were asked to select and write down your personal objectives for learning about cultural assessments and culturally appropriate nursing diagnoses. Please review those objectives now.

1. To what extent have you met each objective that you selected from the list of objectives? _____
   _____

2. To what extent have you met the personal objectives that you listed separately? _____
   _____

3. What new objectives have you developed since you began reading this Unit? _____
   _____

Exercise Two: Evaluating Your Personal Responses to Conducting Cultural Assessments and Writing Culturally Appropriate Nursing Diagnoses

Now that you have studied this unit, and have probably had some clinical experience assessing patients and developing nursing diagnoses, redo Exercise Two from this unit's self-assessment section. Choose the answer that best describes your point of view now that you have finished this unit and have recorded your experiences in your diary.

	Agree	Neutral	Disagree
I should be able to learn how to perform a competent cultural assessment within a few months.	_____	_____	_____
I do not need to culturally assess a patient from my own culture.	_____	_____	_____
I need to ask my patients what they believe has caused their illness.	_____	_____	_____
I think that most people do self-care before seeking medical care.	_____	_____	_____
I am comfortable writing nursing diagnoses for patients from other cultures.	_____	_____	_____
I understand how to use nursing diagnoses.	_____	_____	_____
When writing nursing diagnoses, I frequently ask myself: Could I be wrong?	_____	_____	_____
I believe that writing nursing diagnoses is a waste of time.	_____	_____	_____
Some of the nursing diagnoses I have used do not seem to make any sense.	_____	_____	_____
Patients should be involved in their nursing diagnoses and treatment.	_____	_____	_____
Nursing diagnoses must be applied equally to every patient, regardless of culture.	_____	_____	_____

Exercise Three: Reviewing Your *Transcultural Interaction Diary*

1. What positive experiences (if any) have you had in conducting cultural assessments and writing culturally appropriate nursing diagnoses?

_____

2. What negative experiences (if any) have you had in conducting cultural assessments and writing culturally appropriate nursing diagnoses?

_____

3. What difficulties or challenges have you faced as you assessed patients from other cultures?

_____

_____

What do you feel caused those difficulties?

_____

_____

What did you do to overcome those difficulties or challenges?

_____

_____

4. What difficulties or challenges have you faced as you identified, documented, and used culturally appropriate nursing diagnoses?

_____

_____

What do you feel caused those difficulties?

_____

_____

What did you do to overcome those difficulties or challenges?

_____

_____

Exercise Four: Evaluating Your Readiness for (a) Conducting Cultural Assessments and (b) Identifying, Using, and Sharing Culturally Appropriate Nursing Diagnoses

Write a brief response to these questions, which are drawn from topics discussed in Chapters 7 through 10.

1. The cultural assessment is vitally important because it helps to ensure that health care providers:
   a. _____
   b. _____

2. *Cultural blind spot syndrome* is defined as _____

_____

3. Nurses appear to pass through five distinct stages before they become experts at conducting cultural assessments. These stages are:

   a. _____

   b. _____

   c. _____

   d. _____

   e. _____

   f. _____

4. Fong's CONFHER model provides a systemic framework for organizing cultural assessment questions and answers. CONFHER stands for:

   C _____ Example: _____

   O _____ Example: _____

   N _____ Example: _____

   F _____ Example: _____

   H _____ Example: _____

   E _____ Example: _____

   R _____ Example: _____

5. The *Explanatory Model* (EM) is defined as _____
   _____

6. If your assessment indicates that your patient is also doing self-care, you should _____
   _____

7. A *genogram* is _____
   _____

   Components of a genogram are: _____
   _____

8. List four ways in which a patient's culture can change the way a nurse identifies and uses a nursing diagnosis.

   a. _____

   b. _____

   c. _____

   d. _____

9. Record at least three ways nurses can communicate culturally appropriate nursing diagnoses to peers and other members of the health care team.

   a. _____

   b. _____

   c. _____

   d. _____

10. Identify at least one transcultural communication concern with each of the following nursing diagnosis labels.

    Verbal communication, Impaired:

    _____

    Thought processes, Disturbed:

    _____

    Noncompliance:

    _____

    Knowledge deficient:

    _____

    Social interaction, Impaired:

    _____

    Powerlessness:

    _____

11. Leininger identified six concerns regarding NANDA's nursing taxonomy. These six concerns are:

    a. _____

    b. _____

    c. _____

    d. _____

    e. _____

    f. _____

    What gaps in the current NANDA nursing diagnosis list have you discovered? _____

    _____

    _____

12. What do you see as your professional role regarding the diagnosis of culturally diverse patients?

_____

_____

13. What communication skills are most likely to help you formulate, implement, document, and share culturally appropriate nursing diagnoses?

_____

_____

UNIT FOUR

Using Transcultural Communication Skills to Plan and Implement Care

UNIT FOUR
ASSESSMENT

ASSESSING YOUR TRANSCULTURAL COMMUNICATION SKILLS IN PLANNING AND IMPLEMENTING CARE

Exercise One: Assessing How Comfortable You Feel When Planning and Implementing Care for Patients from Diverse Cultures

Planning care, teaching patients, relieving pain, consoling the dying, and assisting grieving relatives and friends are all very important nursing duties. It takes intense study and years of practice to feel truly comfortable when communicating with patients from diverse cultures who need instruction, guidance, and counsel.

This exercise will help you to assess your current level of comfort with these transcultural interactions. The following statements contain assignments that you might receive as you work with patients from diverse cultures. Using the following five levels of comfort, rate how you feel about performing each assignment.

- Level 1: I feel very uncomfortable.
- Level 2: I feel rather uncomfortable.
- Level 3: I feel fairly comfortable.
- Level 4: I feel comfortable.
- Level 5: I feel very comfortable.

1. *Assignment:* Talk with a patient about his financial and home situation—two factors that can influence your plan of care. **1 2 3 4 5**

2. *Assignment:* Explain to a Japanese patient who regularly uses soy sauce and other similar flavorings that he must reduce the sodium in his diet to control his congestive heart failure. **1 2 3 4 5**

3. *Assignment:* Negotiate a biomedical plan of care with a patient from a culture that does not totally accept biomedical practices.

    1 2 3 4 5

4. *Assignment:* Witness a patient's signing of an *Informed Consent* before a major procedure. **1 2 3 4 5**

5. *Assignment:* Develop clear, realistic, and measurable learning objectives for a patient who needs to learn about his medications, diet, rest, and activity schedule before going home. **1 2 3 4 5**

6. *Assignment:* Teach a patient a procedure such as changing a dressing or self-administration of insulin. **1 2 3 4 5**

7. *Assignment:* Work closely with an interpreter to teach a patient with limited English proficiency about his diet and medications.

   1 2 3 4 5

8. *Assignment:* Counsel a patient with chronic pain who is from an emotive culture: for example, the Italian culture. **1 2 3 4 5**

9. *Assignment:* Counsel and console a dying patient and his family who are observing cultural and religious rituals with which you are unfamiliar.

   1 2 3 4 5

Exercise Two: Assessing Your Point of View toward Transcultural Nursing Situations That Involve Planning, Teaching, Counseling, and Consoling

How do you feel about using transcultural communication techniques to plan care, explain, teach, and counsel patients from diverse cultures? Do you feel that it is very important to consider the patient's cultural background when planning and providing care and instruction? Or do you feel that cultural considerations are much less important than other aspects of nursing care? Select the answers that best describe your point of view *now*, before you proceed with the chapters in this unit. There is no scoring for these questions.

1. When planning care for patients from diverse cultures, you should
   a. make every effort to preserve the patients' cultural practices
   b. consider the patients' cultural practices, but make the biomedical aspects of the patients' care plan your major priority
   c. convince the patients that they should follow the medical and nursing care plan for their own good
   d. let the patients manage their own care as much as possible

2. A patient who refuses to follow a biomedical plan of care
   a. needs to have logical reasons for his refusal to follow the plan
   b. is being unreasonable and noncompliant
   c. is observing his legal and constitutional rights
   d. is recklessly endangering his health and should be scheduled for a psychiatric consult

3. When teaching patients from diverse cultures
   a. I try to provide the same information in the same way, regardless of a patient's cultural background.
   b. I try to consider each patient's special learning needs and limitations that are related to his or her culture or lack of proficiency in English.
   c. I don't believe that it is possible to write measurable learning objectives for patients.
   d. I realize that sometimes it is necessary to negotiate with patients and must adapt my teaching plan to their cultural views and daily patterns.

4. When caring for patients from diverse cultures who are experiencing pain
   a. I realize that some patients are stoic in their response to pain, whereas other patients are emotive.
   b. It is difficult to evaluate a patient's pain when the person responds in a stoic manner and refuses to acknowledge that the pain exists.
   c. It is difficult to work with patients who scream and cry when in pain.
   d. The patient's own description of his or her pain is often inaccurate.

5. When caring for patients from diverse cultures who are dying
   a. I try to accept each patient's cultural values and behavior patterns regarding dying and death.
   b. I find it difficult to deal with the dying patient's family, when their continuous presence makes it hard for me to provide care.
   c. I don't know what to say when family members express their grief to me after the patient's death.
   d. I don't feel that I have the experience to counsel a bereaved family from another culture.

Exercise Three: Using Your *Transcultural Interaction Diary*

1. Before reading the chapters in this unit, please set up the following four new sections in your diary. Each section should address your feelings, thoughts, activities, and experiences while: (a) planning care for patients from diverse cultures, (b) developing and implementing a teaching plan, (c) caring for patients in pain, and (d) assisting patients and families as they work their way through the patient's death experience.

2. Start recording in your diary *now*, before studying this unit.

3. Before reading Chapter 13, recall and make a note of the times when you have *planned care* for patients from different cultures. Were these experiences positive, neutral, or negative? In each case, how did the patient respond to your plan? Did the patient totally accept your plan, accept only parts of your plan, or reject your plan? If a patient from another culture did reject your plan, how did it make you feel? Concerned? Upset? Angry? Insulted? How did you respond to the patient? Did you try to convince him that he was wrong? Or did you try to negotiate and compromise with the patient? How did you resolve this situation?

4. Next write down any memorable *teaching experiences*. Have you had an opportunity to develop a formal teaching plan? What types of patient teaching have you done? Informal teaching at the bedside? Group presentations? Demonstrations of procedures? Do you feel comfortable teaching patients about their care? If you have had any very positive or negative experiences while teaching, write them down now. Take a few minutes and analyze each teaching experience and your feelings about it.

5. As you study Chapter 13, use your diary to record new experiences as you develop care plans and teaching plans for patients from diverse cultures. Use the transcultural communication techniques suggested in Chapter 13 to help you present your plans to your patients and to negotiate compromises if necessary. If possible, try to follow your patients' progress even after they leave your health care facility. Try to stay in touch with patients through phone calls, letters, or home visits. Keep a record in your diary of how your patients are utilizing the health care information that you taught them.

6. Before reading Chapter 14, recall and write down your experiences with patients from diverse cultures who were experiencing *pain*. How did these patients respond to their pain? In a stoic manner? In an emotive manner? In each case, how did you evaluate your patient's pain? What did you do to relieve the patient's pain? In general, were these experiences positive or negative? Take a few minutes and analyze each experience and your feelings.

7. Next write down any experiences that you have had with patients from diverse cultures who were *dying*. Were these experiences positive or negative? Did these patients and their families seem to accept death, or did they refuse to confront death? What cultural and religious practices did the dying patient and family observe? Did these practices offer solace and comfort? Were you able to accept these practices and the

patient's dying wishes? What were you able to do to counsel and console the patient and family? Were your actions successful? If so, why?

8. As you study Chapter 14, continue to record your experiences and feelings as you work with patients who are in pain or who are dying. Practice using the transcultural communication techniques presented in this chapter, and then record which techniques were successful for you and which were not. Also, learn all you can about the various ways in which people from different cultures may respond to pain, death, and grief. For example, Asians tend to respond to pain in a stoic manner, whereas Italians are more emotive. Note in your diary if your patient's response to pain or critical illness was more in keeping with his or her culture or with mainstream American culture.

9. As you work with your diary, remember to keep it in a private place. Your diary contains a record of your personal experiences with patients from different cultures. No one should have access to your diary, unless you choose to share it with someone you trust.

CHAPTER 13

Using Transcultural Communication to Plan Care, Explain, and Instruct

KEY TERMS

- Advance Directives
- Alternative Resources
- Care Plan
- Compliance
- Cultural Demands
- Culturally Generated Feelings
- Culture Brokering
- Education by Appropriate Analogy

- Financial Resources
- Informed Consent
- Knowledge Deficit
- Language Barrier
- Learning Needs
- LEARN Model
- Nonadherence
- Patient Self-Determination Act

OBJECTIVES

After completing this chapter, you should be able to:

- Use transcultural communication skills when planning care for patients from other cultures.
- Recognize obstacles that you should discuss with patients from other cultures before finalizing their care plan.
- Develop a care plan that is sensitive to the patient's cultural needs.

- Appreciate the impact of the Patient Self-Determination Act on the rights of patients to make informed decisions about their own care.

- Identify the patient's learning style and use the transcultural teaching method that is most appropriate.

- Teach patients from other cultures how to self-administer medications and assist with or perform prescribed procedures at home.

- Recognize the reasons why patients from other cultures may not comply with your care plan and self-care instructions.

INTRODUCTION

Transcultural communication plays a vital role in all aspects of the nursing process. Transcultural communication skills are needed not only for assessing and diagnosing patients from different cultures but also for planning, implementing, and evaluating their care and learning needs. The use of transcultural communication techniques to gather patient information and design culturally appropriate nursing diagnoses was discussed in Chapters 11 and 12.

This chapter, which consists of two parts, spotlights planning and implementation. Part one focuses on using transcultural communication to develop care plans that will be acceptable to patients from diverse cultures. Part two concentrates on implementing care plans. It explores how to use transcultural communication techniques to teach patients about their care and evaluate the results.

USING TRANSCULTURAL COMMUNICATION TO PLAN CARE

From your study of the nursing process, you already know that planning a patient's care is the crucial third step of the process. In general, developing a **care plan** involves

1. Establishing priorities based on the nursing diagnoses.

2. Developing outcomes with deadlines or target dates for their completion.

3. Developing a plan of action.

4. Writing the care plan.

5. Implementing and evaluating the care plan (Bolander, 1994).

The American Nurses Association (ANA) has established measurement criteria for patient care plans. To meet ANA standards, a care plan must:

- Be individualized to the patient's condition or needs.
- Be developed with the patient and significant others when possible.
- Reflect current nursing practice.
- Be documented.
- Provide for continuity of care.

To develop an acceptable care plan for patients with whom you share cultural values can be quite a challenge. Developing a care plan for patients from different cultures takes the planning process one giant step further. The care plan must not only meet the patient's needs, but it must also acknowledge and respect the patient's beliefs and values. The following sections describe the role of culture in care planning and provide some specific transcultural communication techniques that will help you develop a plan that your patient will accept and follow.

General Considerations

To develop a successful care plan for a patient from another culture, you will need to first conduct a thorough cultural assessment (see Chapter 11). It is important to ask patients about their religious beliefs, family relationships, prior hospital experiences, dietary choices, and health beliefs and practices. The more you learn about your patient's cultural background and preferences, the more likely it is that your patient will find your plan acceptable.

Leininger outlined the following three major approaches to planning care for patients from different cultural backgrounds (Jackson, 1993).

1. Make every effort to *preserve* the patient's cultural health beliefs and practices that are beneficial. Acupuncture, acupressure, and some herbal medicines are examples of cultural practices that may help patients feel better.

2. *Adapt* or *adjust* the patient's cultural beliefs and practices to fit your care plan, provided they are not harmful. The wearing of amulets, certain religious practices, or use of other types of healers in conjunction with biomedical interventions are examples of practices that neither harm nor necessarily help patients. Let your patients know that they are free to observe these cultural and religious practices, but they should also follow their biomedical care plan.

3. Try to *repattern* cultural beliefs and practices that could potentially harm the patient's health. For example, Asians traditionally consume foods and flavorings that are high in sodium, such as soy sauce. These food items are dangerous for people with hypertension and heart disease. Although the patient may not be willing to completely give up soy sauce, you may be able to persuade the person to use a reduced sodium soy sauce preparation.

Unfortunately, despite your best intentions, care planning may not always proceed smoothly. Patients and their families may not understand or accept biomedical practices or your proposed interventions, and thus fail to follow through on your plan. When your patient's health beliefs and practices are at odds with biomedical beliefs and practices, you will need to *negotiate* your care plan through the process of **culture brokering**. (See Chapter 10 for more details.) Culture brokering is defined as "the act of bridging, linking, or mediating between groups or persons through the process of reducing conflict or producing change" (Chalanda, 1995). A good culture broker (1) respects the values of both cultures and their health care systems, (2) is knowledgeable about both cultures, and (3) is able to overcome any existing language barriers, so that everyone clearly understands each other.

Cultural brokering or cultural negotiation can be very useful when working with patients using the healing practice called *coining*. This practice involves the use of a coin rubbed against the skin to create redness and warmth in the skin surface. The belief underlying this practice is that the "cause" of the illness or distress (i.e., spirits) will be able to escape or leave the body through the skin. However, the vigorous rubbing may cause severe skin irritation and breakdown that can commonly be misinterpreted as child abuse. Knowing the cultural basis of coining, the nurse can initiate the negotiation. The nurse may suggest using less vigorous motion when rubbing or, perhaps, covering the coin with a soft material to lessen the friction, thereby diminishing skin irritation. These suggestions will be offered and need to be mutually agreed upon by the client and the health care provider.

The nurse who is a skilled culture broker will try to negotiate with the patient and family when conflicts arise concerning the care plan. The nurse can begin by explaining the biomedical approach to treatment. Next, she can inquire about the patient's health care beliefs, and she can ask the patient how he or she feels the condition should be treated. Without trying to change the patient's beliefs, the nurse should encourage the patient to think of ways to overcome objections to the plan. Whenever possible, it is important to incorporate the patient's suggestions into the nursing care plan.

• • • COMMUNICATION CONSIDERATIONS • • •

The patient who is actively involved in making decisions about the health care is far more likely to cooperate with the nurse's plan of care.

Sometimes, even the most skilled culture broker cannot overcome a patient's resistance to a biomedical plan of care. In such a case, it is easy to become frustrated and angry with the patient. A patient may even be labeled as noncompliant!

Although health professionals may strongly object to a patient's decision to reject their plan of care, the fact is that *all patients have the constitutional right to refuse treatment* without giving reasons. Patients are guaranteed this right under the **Patient Self-Determination Act** (PSDA), which was passed by the U.S. Congress in 1990 and became effective on December 1, 1991.

Since the enactment of the PSDA in 1991, there has been a greater emphasis on obtaining the patient's **informed consent** prior to treatment. The consent process ensures that the patient has received enough information to make an informed decision about interventions recommended by the physician, for example, a surgical procedure (Mailhot, 1997). Through the use of **advance directives** (living will or durable power of attorney), the PSDA also guarantees patients the right to make decisions—in advance—about their care should they become mentally incapacitated. For example, some patients may not want to be kept on life support if they have suffered brain damage (Lim, 1997).

In the words of Ulrich (1994), "The PSDA is a powerful tool in the United States to express society's commitment to personal and cultural diversity and to protect it against violation by those who might think they have a privileged place in society that allows them to dictate to others what is in their best interest."

When a patient refuses to follow the plan of care that you and the physician feel is best, what can you do? The first thing you must do is recognize that patients have a right to make health-related decisions that are based on their cultural beliefs and values; after all, it is their life. On the other hand, you do not have to agree with your patient's decisions, and you can voice your objections. Nevertheless, you will ultimately need to accept your patient's choices. As Charonko points out, "As caregivers our role is to help [patients] live as productively as they can within their own choices. Our role then becomes one of facilitating their efforts to find the resources they will need to meet their goals" (Charonko, 1992).

Specific Techniques

Before beginning to develop your care plan, carefully review all the information about your patient that you have gathered during the assessment process. Using your transcultural communication skills, you can then enlarge upon this information as you prepare your care plan. Basic steps in transcultural care planning are as follows:

1. Review the patient's *preferences for care* and then include them in your care plan whenever possible. For example, a patient is more likely to follow a prescribed diet if it includes at least some favorite items.

2. Review the patient's *cultural preferences* and make every effort to accommodate those preferences in your plan. A lack of accommodation on your part can lead to resentful resistance by the patient and frustration for you. To achieve accommodation, phrase your plan in terms that are consistent with the patient's cultural background. You also need to develop a plan that will work within the patient's normal cultural environment; for example, within home and work environments.

   Example: Members of some cultural groups believe in the concept that heat and cold are associated with illness. A Pakistani patient who had a cold refused to drink the cold juices the nurse offered. It did not make sense to him to treat cold with cold. If a patient seems reluctant to take the medications, fluids, or foods that are in his care plan, you might ask the patient if he believes in hot or cold notions of illness. The patient's decisions regarding what to eat or drink may be based on those beliefs.

3. Address **language barriers** in your care plan. For instance, when you are caring for a patient whose native language is not English, include this nursing diagnosis in your plan:

   Impaired verbal communications related to limited ability to speak or understand the dominant language of the health care delivery system.

   On the care plan, you will want to indicate what resources or strengths the person has that will help reduce the language barrier. For instance:

   • Patient can read simple English phrases.
   • Patient understands some basic words in English.

- Patient can follow short, simple instructions spoken in English.
- Patient relies on daughter to interpret. Daughter is available in the evenings for interpretation.

4. Include the patient's *family and significant others* in your care plan. Who in the family makes the major decisions? Which family members will be responsible for the patient after discharge? What tasks will these family members be expected to perform? Will family members need any special instructions or training?

   Also, you will want to investigate how the patient's illness has affected family relationships. For example, in extended families the patient's illness may have disrupted that person's role (or roles) within the family, such as family head, primary breadwinner, or primary caregiver. After recovery, the patient may need to be reintegrated into the usual family role. If so, you will want to address that process in your care plan.

5. Review the patient's *religious beliefs*. In your care plan, note if the patient wishes to observe certain rituals or religious dietary requirements. For example, Catholic patients may want to receive daily communion, whereas Orthodox Jewish patients will want to observe Jewish dietary laws.

6. Consider the patient's *level of knowledge* concerning the disease process and its treatment. If the patient is not knowledgeable, you will want to block out ample time to instruct the patient about the diagnosis, medications, procedures, and home care.

7. Discuss the **financial resources** that the patient must have to comply with a prescribed regimen. If the patient appears to have very limited financial means, ask the following:
   - Do you receive coupons or vouchers for getting your prescribed medications?
   - Have you contacted a local agency for temporary financial assistance?
   - Has anyone referred you to an agency that can provide temporary financial assistance?
   - Has our dietitian suggested foods that you can afford? Can you find these items where you shop?

8. Discuss any *other obstacles* that the patient faces, such as a lack of child care or transportation.

Example: A 14-year-old Alaskan Native American patient was discharged from an urban Northwestern hospital with her 3-day-old baby. The nurse instructed the young mother to return to the hospital laboratory the next day to have her baby's bilirubin level checked. However, upon further questioning, the nurse learned that the mother had been in the city for only two weeks, had never ridden on a bus, and had no bus tokens or money for a taxi. The nurse had the mother go to social services, where she received a bus pass.

···· COMMUNICATION CONSIDERATIONS ····

Caution: When questioning a patient about available resources, be careful not to simply assume that the patient will have problems coping because of youth or poverty.

On the other hand, a 26-year-old mother of four children in a large city was instructed to bring her daughter to the public health department for a dental checkup. Although the mother had already spent her state Aid to Families with Dependent Children grant money, she was resourceful. The mother walked to a social service agency to get bus tokens, which allowed her to keep her daughter's dental appointment.

9. Once you have identified obstacles, look for **alternative resources** available in the patient's family and community and help your patient use those resources. For example, you might ask the patient, "Do you have a relative who lives nearby who can watch your children for a couple of hours while you come to the clinic for treatment?"

10. Be aware of any **cultural demands** that the patient faces at home that may compete with important health care needs. When doing discharge planning, ask the patient what activities a typical day includes and what role(s) the patient plays in the family.

Example: A visiting nurse was surprised to find her 68-year-old Salvadoran patient standing over a stove cooking. The patient had recently been discharged after surgery to correct an intestinal obstruction. Because the care plan did not state that the woman cared for her three grandchildren while her daughter worked, the nurse had expected to find the patient resting. The nurse rewrote the care plan and made arrangements for social services to provide a chore person who could come to the house every day while the patient recuperated.

11. Identify any **culturally generated feelings** (e.g., feelings of guilt or shame) that may undermine a patient's willingness to follow a health care plan.

> **Example:** A white middle-class family nurse practitioner (FNP) informed a 70-year-old Hispanic male with adult-onset diabetes that he needed to eat a prescribed diet that included more vegetables and fewer tortillas and beans. During a follow-up appointment, the FNP discovered that the patient was not following the diet. Careful questioning by the FNP revealed that (1) the patient lived with his son and daughter-in-law, who did all the food preparation; (2) the daughter-in-law had no idea that the patient was to follow a therapeutic diet; and (3) the patient was ashamed to admit he needed to diet, especially because it would be more costly for the family to provide the different food.
>
> In reviewing her notes on Hispanic culture, the FNP noted that studies by Albert in 1986 indicated that Hispanics are more interpersonally oriented than whites and that Hispanic behavior is more frequently related to feelings of shame than is white behavior. Recognizing these cultural differences, the FNP involved the son and daughter-in-law in the plan of care. She also had the dietitian write out suggestions for buying and preparing the prescribed foods at low cost. On her next visit, the FNP was relieved to find that the entire family was enjoying meals that included more vegetables and other healthful foods.

12. Respect culturally influenced practices and patterns of behavior that are related to *gender*. For example, female patients from Hispanic or Arabic cultures may feel very uncomfortable in the presence of male care providers. In such cases, you might note in your care plan: "Assign female nurses" or "Have a female assistant accompany male health care providers."

13. Above all, recognize your patient's concerns and address them in your care plan.

Patients may view their condition differently from the nurse and they may have different concerns. Some patients perceive the social and psychologic ramifications of their disorder as more important than the medical ramifications that concern nurses.

Example: A nurse in the arthritis clinic of an urban medical center spent a great deal of time discussing possible medication reactions with her patients. However, her elderly patients were primarily worried about how they would care for themselves if they lost their mobility. Because the nurse failed to address the patients' concerns, they often left the clinic feeling that their real needs had been ignored.

• • • COMMUNICATION CONSIDERATIONS • • •

Communication between nurse and patient must be a two-way process. Although you need to discuss your concerns with patients, it is equally important to listen to their concerns and plan care accordingly.

USING TRANSCULTURAL COMMUNICATION TO EXPLAIN AND INSTRUCT

Transcultural communication provides nurses with a powerful tool for implementing their nursing care plans. By using transcultural communication techniques, nurses can provide patients from diverse cultures with the vital information they must have to act as partners in their care.

Teaching the patient about the care plan can be done on an impromptu basis. For example, while administering medications to a patient, you can explain the benefits the person will receive from the prescribed drugs. You can instruct a patient in what to expect during a special procedure. While serving a patient a special diet, you can discuss which foods are permitted on the diet, which are not permitted, and why.

Patient teaching may also be conducted in a more formal manner by using and implementing a written teaching plan. Although providing patient education has always been an important nursing responsibility, the patient education programs were primarily developed by white nurses to meet the needs of white patients, or they were modified to meet the needs of ethnic patients by including a token amount of cultural information (Tripp-Reimer & Afifi, 1989). Only since the 1990s have nurses really tried to address the learning needs of patients from diverse cultures.

The following sections contain basic transcultural teaching principles and special techniques that you can use when instructing ethnic patients.

General Considerations

To successfully instruct patients from diverse cultures, the first thing you must do is establish rapport with your patients by using the transcultural communication techniques described throughout this book. You can use these techniques to do impromptu teaching and to develop planned patient teaching programs.

To develop a planned teaching/learning program, you will need to adapt the five steps of the nursing process to the teaching/learning process as follows: (1) Assess the patient's learning needs; (2) diagnose the patient's knowledge deficits; (3) develop a teaching plan; (4) implement your teaching plan; and (5) evaluate your patient's progress, making adjustments to your teaching plan as necessary. The sections that follow describe these important steps.

Assess and Diagnose Patient's Learning Needs. Before you can proceed to teach, you must first identify your patient's **learning needs**. For instance, does the patient know anything about the biomedical health care system and how it works? What does the patient already know about the disorder? Does the person want to learn more about this illness? Does the patient need specific information about a surgery or procedure before signing an Informed Consent Form? Do you need to discuss the benefits of a special diet or warn the person about possible side effects from medications? Do you need to demonstrate the procedure that the person or significant others will have to perform after discharge?

Note that patients from different ethnic groups may differ in their learning needs. For example, Chinese American patients may want you to explain the cause of illness. Jewish patients may want to know about the actions and side effects of their medications in detail.

Next you need to consider the person's *readiness to learn*. Does the person seem motivated to learn? Does the patient want to understand how medications and biomedical treatments will help? On the other hand, is the person too exhausted or in too much pain to concentrate on your explanations? Is the patient too anxious to remember your instructions?

> ### ● ● ● COMMUNICATION CONSIDERATIONS ● ● ●
>
> Before beginning your teaching sessions, make certain that your patient is rested and free of pain. If the patient appears frightened or anxious, talk with the person about worries and concerns before attempting to teach.

Finally, does the patient have any *limitations* that could interfere with learning? For instance, does the patient have limited English proficiency? Is this a person of limited financial resources who is unable to purchase foods for a special diet or buy medications and thus sees no reason to remember your instructions? Will the patient be burdened with work and family responsibilities after discharge that will limit the time available to follow your schedule for rest and exercise?

> ### ● ● ● COMMUNICATION CONSIDERATIONS ● ● ●
>
> Try to work out ways to resolve the patient's limitations before starting to teach. For patients with limited English proficiency, arrange for an interpreter to be present during your teaching sessions. Have a social worker meet with patients who have serious financial problems. Ask for the family's help when patients feel too burdened with responsibilities to follow your instructions and take care of their health.

After you have completed your assessment, you should next establish *culturally appropriate nursing diagnoses*. Nursing diagnoses that are linked with the patient's learning needs are usually worded as **knowledge deficits** (e.g., knowledge deficit related to low-calorie diet). However, as Chapter 12 points out, this use of *knowledge deficit* is often inaccurate. A knowledge deficit (a lack of knowledge) is the *reason* a problem exists, and thus it should appear in the "related to" part of the nursing diagnosis. The term *knowledge deficit* should then be followed with a statement that pinpoints the specific subject matter that the patient needs to learn to correct a problem. For example:

- Altered nutrition, more than body requirements related to knowledge deficit of low-calorie foods and beverages.

- High risk for fluid volume excess related to knowledge deficit of low-sodium diet.

- High risk for constipation related to knowledge deficit of high-fiber foods and adequate fluid intake.

Develop a Teaching Plan. The next step is to develop a teaching plan. Your teaching plan should be a carefully organized, written presentation that specifies what you want your patient to learn and how you plan to present the information. For instance, you may want your patient to learn about how to purchase and prepare the foods on a special diet. Or you may want to prepare for discharge by teaching the patient how to change dressings at home. Remember to invite the patient's family members to your teaching sessions. Your teaching program will be most successful if the patient's family understands how important it is for the patient to follow the prescribed treatment regimen.

Your method of teaching should be based on the patient's *preferred learning style*, which, in turn, may be grounded in the person's cultural background. Many patients prefer to learn with written materials prepared in a language that they can read and understand with ease. Patients from cultures that are characterized by a strong oral tradition may prefer educational films presented in their language. They may also appreciate a group setting where members of the group talk about their experiences and act as peer educators (Tripp-Reimer & Afifi, 1989). Performing demonstrations and asking for return demonstrations is the best way to teach procedures.

Education by appropriate analogy provides another method for presenting information. According to Nichter and Nichter (1996), education by analogy is "not a new method of education but rather a use of the familiar to explain the new." They further explain that:

> a good analogy is like a plow which can prepare a population's field of associations for planting a new idea. If the field of associations is not adequately plowed to accommodate new ideas, it is difficult for such ideas to take root. Equal effort needs to be put into preparing the field, improving the plow, and perfecting the spread of seed.

Here is an analogical message that was developed to teach families in the Philippines birth control by using an intrauterine device (IUD).

> The IUD is like a fence which the farmer places around his fields to prevent animals from entering and destroying the garden. Placed inside a woman, an IUD prevents her from getting pregnant by preventing the seed from taking root in the uterus.

During the planning period, you will also want to develop some *learning objectives* for your patients. Learning objectives should be clear and realistic. You should also be able to measure your patient's progress. The following are examples of learning objectives for Mr. Gonzales, a 65-year-old Hispanic male who has just been diagnosed with congestive heart failure.

- *Objective 1:* By the end of the first learning session, Mr. Gonzales will be able to explain why it is important for him to eat low-sodium foods and drink low-sodium beverages.

- *Objective 2:* By the end of the second learning session, Mr. Gonzales will be able to list the foods, seasonings, beverages, and over-the-counter medications that are not allowed on his low-sodium diet.

- *Objective 3:* By the end of the third learning session, Mr. Gonzales will be able to list foods, seasonings, and beverages that are low in sodium. He and his wife will have identified markets where they purchase low-sodium items.

- *Objective 4:* Before being discharged, Mr. Gonzales and his wife will have met with the dietitian, who will assist them in modifying favorite recipes by substituting low-sodium ingredients and seasonings.

- *Objective 5:* During the first home visit, Mr. Gonzales and his wife will have been able to show the nurse the low-sodium items they have purchased and are now using for meal preparation.

•••• COMMUNICATION CONSIDERATIONS ••••

For learning to take place, the patient must believe in your proposed learning objectives as much as you do. For the greatest success, the patient needs to be personally involved in the planning stage of your educational program.

Implement the Teaching Plan and Evaluate the Patient's Progress.
Once you have completed your teaching plan and obtained your patient's cooperation, you can put your plan into action. You will need to schedule learning sessions with your patient and family. If the patient has difficulty with English, have an interpreter present during your sessions. It also helps to invite *resource people* to assist you with your teaching. For example, the dietitian can talk with patients about special diets; a physical therapist can teach patients how to do active range-of-motion exercises, and a pharmacist can explain the side effects of medications.

Once the patient goes home, it is very important to follow up your teaching with telephone calls, home visits, letters, or return clinic visits. If you are not able to perform follow-up duties yourself, refer the person to the appropriate individuals who can continue to supervise the patient's health education. For long-term follow-up, health care facilities sometimes send health education questionnaires to patients.

The final step in the teaching/learning process is to *evaluate* the extent to which the patient has met the learning objectives and has sustained a change in behavior. Changing behaviors takes time, and change is often impeded by occasional setbacks. Food habits in particular are very difficult to change.

When a patient experiences setbacks, it is important to reassess the patient and then evaluate your teaching plan, update it, and implement it again. Because learning is a lifelong endeavor, it may take patients many months or even years to make permanent changes in their health-related behaviors.

To summarize, the **LEARN model** (Figure 13-1) developed by Berlin and Fowkes (1983) emphasizes the major steps that are involved in teaching patients from diverse cultures about their health, illnesses, medications, and treatments.

LEARN MODEL

1. **L**isten and ask questions to assess the patient's term for illness as well as what the patient believes is causing the illness.

2. **E**xplain (using simple terms) what the patient needs to understand about his or her illness. Also explain the reasons for your nursing interventions.

3. **A**cknowledge that the patient's views may differ from your own. You probably adhere to the biomedical model of care, whereas the patient may believe in the traditional model. Take care not to devalue the patient's views.

4. **R**ecommend what you would like your patient to do. For example, practice drawing insulin or practice changing a dressing.

5. **N**egotiate with the patient and adapt your recommendations to the patient's views and daily patterns. Have the patient assume some control over aspects of the therapeutic plan.

Figure 13-1 LEARN Model. Adapted from Berlin & Fowkes, 1983.

Specific Techniques

Learning about prescribed medications, new procedures, self-care activities, and important lifestyle changes within the busy and sometimes impersonal hospital environment can be confusing and upsetting for any patient. But such illness-related experiences are more confusing, stressful, and even frightening when the patient is from another culture. The best way to eliminate your patient's confusion and fear of the new and unknown is to use transcultural communication techniques. Specific techniques for teaching patients from other cultures include the following:

1. Treat patients as individuals first, while remembering that each patient is a member of a cultural group.

2. Follow the general principles of transcultural communication and instruction that were discussed in the preceding sections.

3. Establish rapport with your patient. Patients are more likely to learn from you if they like and trust you.

4. Use the patient's primary language if possible, but have an interpreter present during your teaching sessions when necessary.

5. Before beginning your explanations and instructions, discuss the patient's cultural perspective on illness and therapy. By acknowledging the patient's cultural attitudes, you will be able to provide information that the patient will understand and accept. As a result, the patient will be more willing to make health care choices that you both consider beneficial.

6. When giving instructions, avoid shouting at the patient. Instead, speak softly and clearly. Your tone of voice should be soothing and convey your intent to help.

7. Reduce the noise level in the patient's room so that the patient can concentrate on what you are saying. Recognize that the sound of alarms and monitors can disturb patients, especially those who do not understand the purpose of sophisticated hospital equipment.

8. Try to avoid rushing. You can increase the patient's level of comfort and readiness to receive and provide information if you can convey that you have time to listen. Remember that communication can be potent therapy.

9. Use simple sentences and ask questions that are brief and to the point. Do not say, "Did you take all of your medicines today or did you miss some?" Say rather, "Which medications did you take today?"

10. Repeat instructions, restating them in different words. For example, "Swallow one of these pills every hour until they are all gone.

Swallow a pill at 7:00 AM, 8:00 AM, 9:00 AM, and so on until you have swallowed all of the pills."

11. Use common but specific expressions: *swallow* rather than *take*; *bleeding* or *pus* or *liquid* rather than *discharge*. Avoid using idioms such as *better than nothing* or *start from scratch*.

12. Whenever possible, explain the reason for the patient's symptoms before discussing a medication, intervention, or procedure. For example, when treating a patient with congestive heart failure, try saying:

> Right now your heart isn't able to pump out enough blood to give your body the oxygen and nutrition it needs. This is why you feel so tired. You also have fluid in your lungs, which is making it hard for you to breathe. We're going to give you a daily dose of a medicine called digitalis. Digitalis will help your heart pump better, which will help your blood circulate better. We're also going to give you a water pill. This water pill, or diuretic, will get rid of the extra fluid in your lungs so that you can breathe more easily.

13. Take into account the patient's explanation of why the illness developed and how it might be treated (see the discussion of the explanatory model in Chapter 11). For example:

> I see in your history that your heart problems developed after your son died. You said that you feel like your heart has been damaged by grief. I notice that you are Roman Catholic and that you have been going to Mass every day since your son died. If you would like, I can arrange to have the priest come and visit you daily. We also have a person here in the hospital who helps patients who have recently lost a loved one. Would you like her to stop by?

14. As you explain treatments and procedures, use gestures and simple lay terms. Repeat key words. Avoid technical terminology. Say "your heart attack," not "your myocardial infarction."

15. Explain the steps of procedures in sequence and use progressive statements. "First, place the ice bag on your ankle for 20 minutes. Next, take the ice bag off of your ankle. One hour later, put the ice bag back on your ankle for another 20 minutes."

16. Use diagrams to explain procedures. Patients who are not literate may be confused by two-dimensional diagrams. In these cases, try to use a model if available. For example, use a model of the ear canal to explain how to self-administer eardrops.

17. Use props to demonstrate a procedure. Before giving an injection, first show the patient the equipment (a syringe, needle, alcohol wipes) and then demonstrate how to give an injection. Have the patient do a return demonstration. If the patient has not grasped the procedure, go through the steps of the demonstration and repeat the demonstration.

18. Observe how your patient responds to your instructions. Does he say he understands what you want? Is she able to complete the steps of a procedure? Also, observe the person's body language. Does the patient appear to be upset, confused, withdrawn, or embarrassed? If so, you will want to stop and explore how the patient is feeling.

19. Involve the family in your teaching program. Ask one family member to act as a liaison to the patient's extended family. List the name and phone number of that person in the patient's room, chart, and care plan.

20. Make it easy for the patient and family to contact you for information and instructions once the patient goes home. If you are not able to act as a patient contact, then arrange for another nurse to do so.

21. Recognize that patients from diverse cultures may have legitimate reasons for not complying with your instructions. When patients do not comply, remember that their behavior may be perfectly consistent with cultural values that differ from yours and from the biomedical health care system. Patients who do not comply may also suffer from these nursing diagnoses:

- Decisional conflict related to conflicting cultural values and beliefs.
- Relocation stress syndrome related to cross-cultural migration.
- Impaired verbal communication related to language barriers.

• • • • COMMUNICATION CONSIDERATIONS • • • •

Never try to force change or demand **compliance** from patients. Instead, elicit information from patients that will help you arrive at a mutually agreed-upon care plan and teaching plan. Decide which instructions patients must follow for reasons of safety and then be prepared to negotiate on less crucial items.

When instructing patients who do not speak English or who are not fluent in the language, you will want to perform the following steps in addition to the ones listed previously.

1. Arrange for an interpreter to help you explain procedures and obtain consent.

2. Try to communicate with the patient while you wait for the interpreter to arrive. Never ignore a patient because he or she does not speak your language.

3. Ask a family member to provide additional help with interpreting before surgery or other important procedures. Allow family members to be in the postanesthesia room immediately after the patient regains consciousness.

4. When instructing a patient who does not speak English, frown when you want to signify that the patient should not do something (e.g., no food now). Similarly, nod and smile when you want to reinforce a behavior. When you pour a glass of water, nod and smile as you place the glass in the patient's hand, and then initiate the action of drinking a glass of water.

5. Do use picture cards or a phrase chart (use phonetic pronunciation) as you instruct your patients.

6. If you are caring for a child who does not understand English, you might try short phrases such as, "OK let's go." Try singing children's songs that may be familiar to the child. Use calming gestures and a soothing voice.

7. Assess for comprehension when relaying instructions. Do not assume that the patient's nodding means the patient understands.

8. Look for verbal and nonverbal exchanges between the patient and the family (glances, shaking heads). Do these actions indicate understanding or lack of understanding?

9. Try to locate written educational materials that are in the language of the reader and at the appropriate level of comprehension. For this step, you may need the aid of an interpreter.

The *Transcultural Communication Care Plan* that follows illustrates some of the transcultural communication techniques discussed in this chapter.

TRANSCULTURAL COMMUNICATION CARE PLAN

Communicating with a Hispanic Patient with Heart Failure

Name:	J. Gonzales
Age:	65
Physician:	Dr. Grey
Medical Diagnosis	Congestive heart failure

NURSING DIAGNOSIS

Impaired verbal communication related to limited English proficiency.

ASSESSMENT

- Patient speaks Spanish.
- Patient speaks and understands a few basic words in English.
- Patient's wife speaks and understands more English words than her husband, but is still very limited.
- Patient says over and over "No understand you, no understand you, no understand!"

Expected Outcomes	Interventions	Evaluation
1. Through the interpreter, patient will be able to communicate his symptoms and health concerns.	1. Schedule an interpreter to assist with patient assessment, treatments, and teaching/learning sessions.	1. Mr. Gonzales expressed his symptoms and learning needs through the interpreter.
2. With the aid of the interpreter, patient will be able to give his informed consent to procedures and specify advance directives.	2. Have interpreter explain diagnostic and treatment procedures, informed consent forms, and advance directives.	2. Mr. Gonzales has signed an informed consent for diagnostic procedures. He also made out a living will.

(continues)

Expected Outcomes	Interventions	Evaluation
3. With aid of interpreter, patient and wife will feel prepared to follow the prescribed medical regime at home, and will keep appointments for follow-up clinic visits.	3. Have interpreter assist with discharge planning and scheduling of follow-up clinic appointments.	3. Mr. Gonzales understands his medical regime. His wife has marked down the date in her calendar for their first follow-up clinic visit.

NURSING DIAGNOSIS

Fluid volume excess related to knowledge deficit of low-sodium diet.

ASSESSMENT

- Peripheral edema and neck vein distention present.
- Patient reports eating spicy Mexican foods at home.
- Patient usually asks for salt to sprinkle on his hospital meals.
- Patient says: "No salt? Why not?"

Expected Outcomes	Interventions	Evaluation
1. Patient will be able to understand instructions and ask questions about the new diet.	1. Schedule learning sessions with patient, wife, and interpreter.	1. Mr. Gonzales and wife asked many questions about the new diet.
2. Patient will be able to explain why a low-sodium diet will help his heart condition.	2. Have interpreter explain to patient why it is important to limit sodium intake.	2. Mr. Gonzales was able to explain the purpose of a low-sodium diet in his own words.
3. Patient will be able to list the items that are not allowed on a low-sodium diet.	3. Discuss the foods, beverages, and seasonings that are not allowed on a low-sodium diet.	3. Mr. Gonzales was able to list the items that are not allowed on his low-sodium diet. He seemed to accept these dietary limitations.

(continues)

Expected Outcomes	Interventions	Evaluation
4. Patient will be able to list the foods, beverages, and seasonings that are allowed on a low-sodium diet. He will find out where to purchase these items.	4. Discuss the foods, beverages, and seasonings that are allowed on a low-sodium diet. Explore where the patient and wife can find these items when grocery shopping.	4. Mr. Gonzales was able to list the items that are on his diet. His wife knows where she can find these items in their local super-market.
5. Patient and wife will be able to modify patient's favorite recipes to conform to a low-sodium diet with-out losing "taste appeal."	5. Schedule a meeting with the patient, wife, dietitian, and interpreter. Have wife bring favorite recipes so that dietitian can modify them to conform with patient's low-sodium diet.	5. Mr. Gonzales's wife brought the patient's favorite recipes to the meeting. Mr. Gonzales told interpreter that he will stay on his new diet as long as he can eat his favorite foods, even though they might taste a little different.

NURSING DIAGNOSIS

Nonadherence to clinic appointment schedule related to inability to access public or private transportation.

ASSESSMENT

- Patient discharged from the hospital 3 weeks ago; has missed 3 clinic appointments.

- Patient lives in a rural area that is 50 miles from the clinic.

- Patient and wife do not own a car.

- Using public transportation requires several transfers, and is too exhausting for patient.

- Patient told interpreter: "I am just too tired to wait for all those buses, and too broke to buy a car."

Note: This diagnosis uses the term **nonadherence** rather than *noncompliance*. Nonadherence is less judgmental, and thus a more culturally appropriate nurs-ing diagnosis (see Chapter 12).

(continues)

Expected Outcomes	Interventions	Evaluation
1. Patient and wife will be available for a home visit.	1. Arrange for a meeting at the patient's home. Have patient, wife, interpreter, and social service worker present.	1. Mr. And Mrs. Gonzales seemed glad to meet with us. Patient has been experiencing symptoms of CHF, including orthopnea.
2. Patient will understand that he must have follow-up medical and nursing care to control symptoms.	2. Have interpreter explain the importance of follow-up visits to clinic.	2. Mr. Gonzales told interpreter that he felt very bad about missing his clinic appointments, but he just could not find good transportation.
3. Patient will adhere to the cabulance schedule, and be ready to go to the clinic for appointments.	3. Ask social services to look into having a cabulance pick patient up on clinic days.	3. Mr. Gonzales said to go ahead and make the arrangements for a cabulance to pick him up for his appointments.
4. Patient or his wife will let social services know if he is feeling too ill to go to the clinic.	4. Contact visiting nurse services. Arrange for home visits on days that patient is not up to taking a cabulance to the clinic.	4. Mr. Gonzales was relieved to know that he would receive care at home on days that he was too ill to go to the clinic.
5. Patient will keep clinic appointments once arrangements are made for cabulance.	5. Check with clinic to make sure Mr. Gonzales is keeping appointments.	5. Cabulance was arranged; Mr. Gonzales has kept his last 3 clinic appointments.

REFERENCES

Albert, B. (1986). Review of studies in relational grammar. In D. Perlmutter (Ed.), *Notes on linguistics, 33,* 61–63.

Berlin, E. A., & Fowkes, W. C. (1983). A teaching framework for cross-cultural health care. Application in family practice. *Western Journal of Medicine, 139*(6), 934–938.

Bolander, V. R. (1994). *Sorensen and Luckmann's basic nursing: A psychophysiologic approach* (3rd ed.). Philadelphia: Saunders.

Chalanda, M. (1995). Brokerage in multicultural nursing. *International Nursing Review, 42*(1), 19–22, 26.

Charonko, C. V. (1992). Cultural influences in "noncompliant" behavior and decision making. *Holistic Nursing Practice, 6*(3), 73–138.

Jackson, L. E. (1993). Understanding, eliciting, and negotiating clients' multicultural health beliefs. *Nurse Practitioner, 18*(4), 30–43.

Lim, D. (1997). Culture and advance directives. *American Nephrology Nurses' Association Journal, 24*(1), 69, 97.

Mailhot, C. B. (1997). Culture and consent. *Nursing Management, 28*(3), 48.

Nichter, M., & Nichter, M. (1996). Education by appropriate analogy. In M. Nichter & M. Nichter (Eds.), *Anthropology and international health: Asian case studies* (2nd ed., pp. 400–425). Amsterdam: Gordon and Breach.

Tripp-Reimer, T., & Afifi, L. A. (1989). Cross-cultural perspectives on patient teaching. *Nursing Clinics of North America, 24*(3), 613–619.

Ulrich, L. P. (1994). The Patient Self-Determination Act and cultural diversity. *Cambridge Quarterly of Healthcare Ethics, 3*(3), 410–413.

SUGGESTED READING

Andrews, M. M., & Boyle, J. S. (2002). *Transcultural concepts in nursing care* (6th ed.). Philadelphia: Lippincott.

Bongard, E. S., & Darryl, S. Y. (Ed.) (1993). *Current critical care diagnosis and treatment*. East Norwalk, CT: Appleton & Lange.

Geissler, F. M. (1992). Nursing diagnoses: A study of cultural relevance. *Journal of Professional Nursing, 8*(5), 301–307.

Giger, J. N., & Davidhizar, R. E. (2003). *Transcultural nursing: Assessment and intervention* (4th ed.). St. Louis: Mosby.

Grossman, D. (1996). Cultural dimensions in home health nursing. *American Journal of Nursing, 96*(7), 33–36.

Magnus, M. H. (1996). What's your IQ on cross-cultural nutrition counseling? *The Diabetes Educator, 22*(1), 57–60.

Murphy, F. G., Anderson, R. M., & Lyons, A. E. (1993). Diabetes educators as cultural translators. *The Diabetes Educator, 19*(2), 13–18.

Price, J. L., & Cordell, B. (1994). Cultural diversity and patient teaching. *Journal of Continuing Education in Nursing, 25*(4), 163–166.

Spector, R. E. (2004). *Cultural diversity in health and illness* (6th ed.). Upper Saddle River, NJ: Prentice Hall.

To work with culturally diverse patients, tailor lessons to individual. (1998). *Patient Education Management, 5*(3), 29–32, 44.

CHAPTER 14

Using Transcultural Communication to Assist People Responding to Pain, Grief, Dying, and Death

KEY TERMS

- Appropriate Death
- Death-Accepting
- Death-Defying
- Death-Denying
- Death Phenomenon
- Emotive

- Grief
- Grieving Process
- Pain Phenomenon
- Pain Response
- Stoic

OBJECTIVES

After completing this chapter, you should be able to:

- Describe the significance of using transcultural communication when caring for patients from diverse cultural backgrounds who are experiencing pain.

- Identify barriers to effective transcultural communication between health care professionals and family members whose loved one is dying.

- Describe two broad categories of responses to pain and characteristic features of each.

- Identify nonpharmacologic pain control measures that you can teach to patients to enhance their self-control over the pain.
- Differentiate between different ethnic or cultural groups' responses to pain.
- Identify questions that you can use to elicit the patient's perspective regarding pain.
- Explain three health care practice implications based on responses to pain for each cultural group: Hispanic Americans, Asian Americans, black Americans, white Anglo-Americans, and Native Americans.
- Differentiate between different ethnic or cultural groups' responses to death.
- Describe health care strategies that you can use to effectively assist persons who are grieving.
- Describe five principles that can guide health care professionals during grief counseling.

INTRODUCTION

Pain, dying, death, and grief are powerful universals that eventually affect all people, regardless of their land of birth, culture, or station in life. Although these events produce *similar* responses in people throughout the world (tears, moaning, sighing, screaming out), human responses also *vary*, depending on the person's culture. For example, Asian cultures tend to promote a stoic response to pain and grief, whereas black cultures usually allow emotional expressions of pain and grief. Nurses work intimately with patients and families who are experiencing pain, dying, death, and grief. To support people who are trying to cope with these stressful events, you will need to develop your transcultural communication skills.

Communicating effectively with patients from diverse cultures requires an understanding of the cultural bases for *why* patients and their families react as they do to pain, grief, dying, and death. A lack of sensitivity concerning the effect of culture on a patient's reactions can lead to poor communication, misinterpretation of symptoms, misdiagnoses, and faulty interventions. This chapter addresses how to use transcultural communication to assess, counsel, and console patients from diverse cultures who are suffering and who need your help.

USING TRANSCULTURAL COMMUNICATION TO ASSIST PATIENTS IN PAIN

Pain is a subjective sensation caused by noxious stimuli that signal actual or potential tissue damage. Pain is also a highly personal and private experience influenced by cultural learning, the meaning of the situation, and other factors unique to the individual (Hughes, 1997). An individual's definition of pain, as is that of health and illness, is influenced by personal, social, and cultural experiences.

The Pain Phenomenon

Pain is a universally recognized **phenomenon** and an important area of consideration in health care delivery (Hughes, 1997; Ludwig-Beymer, 1995). Pain probably provides people with the most frequent and compelling reason for seeking health care. People from different cultures may react to pain in different manners because of experiences of pain and suffering. Therefore, knowledge of how different people express pain is essential for the nurse to provide pain relief.

Individuals and cultural groups vary in their **responses** to pain. How people react to pain is influenced by their *perception* of pain. Pain perception, in turn, reflects each individual's attitude toward pain and characteristic way of responding to pain.

The point at which a sensation is first physically perceived and verbalized as painful is called the *pain threshold*. The maximum level of pain a person is willing to endure is called *pain tolerance*. Tolerance to pain is influenced by the individual's cultural background.

Expressions of pain also vary from culture to culture. What are appropriate verbal behavior and body language in response to pain are often dictated by culture. For example, the Japanese culture does not approve of loud verbal expressions of pain. Moreover, *within* each culture, expressions of pain may vary from person to person. For instance, how people express their pain is strongly influenced by their level of assimilation and acculturation into American culture. First- and second-generation descendants of immigrants are likely to respond to pain in conventional ways that are accepted within their parents' or grandparents' traditional culture (Zatzick & Dimsdale, 1990). On the other hand, later generations are less likely to retain traditional attitudes toward pain. There is also a wide range of responses among *subgroups* within the larger ethnic group. For this reason, never assume that all patients from a particular ethnic or cultural group will respond to pain in the same way.

Two broad categories of responses to pain are stoic and emotive responses (Salerno, 1995). Patients who are **stoic** in their response to pain are less expressive verbally and nonverbally, and they rarely complain. Patients who are **emotive** will be quite vocal and will express their pain loudly.

Some reasons for a stoic response to pain include

1. Denial of pain
2. A desire to be the perfect patient
3. Avoiding loss of control
4. Avoiding worrying the family
5. Fear of addiction
6. Fear of overdose and side effects from pain medications
7. Paying a price for past sins and future joys
8. Acceptance of the pain

Some reasons for an emotive response to pain include

1. Fear of the pain
2. A desire for help and fear of not receiving it
3. Anger
4. Grief over loss of role and dignity
5. Exorcism of the pain through the act of crying out
6. Experiencing great pain

In relation to gender, men demonstrate greater stoicism than women; however, research indicates that stoicism decreases with increasing age (Zatzick & Dimsdale, 1990).

Transcultural Differences in Responses to Pain

Mexican Americans come from several diverse subcultural groups, including Hispanics, Puerto Ricans, Spanish Americans, Latin Americans, Latinos, and Chicanos. These different Mexican American subcultures tend to have their own sets of pain-related values, beliefs, and practices.

- Mexican Americans tend to view pain as a necessary part of life and as an indicator of the seriousness of an illness. Mexican Americans believe that enduring sickness, including pain, is a sign of strength. Men often tolerate pain until it becomes unbearable (Klessig, 1992a, b; Villarruel & Ortiz de Montellano, 1992).

- Puerto Rican patients sometimes deny or avoid dealing with pain, but they may exhibit a high anxiety level. Some study findings revealed that Puerto Ricans demonstrated "greater expressiveness of pain, greater interference of pain with daily activities, and higher levels of emotional response to pain" [than their white counterparts] (Gordon, 1997).

- Hispanics and Latin Americans tend not to verbalize complaints of pain.

Asian Americans come from several highly diverse subcultures. In many Asian subcultural groups, pain is considered a serious symptom of illness for which biomedical care is sought. Acupuncture is a popular treatment for many health problems, including pain. Asians generally are quiet in voice and demeanor when in pain (Weber, 1996).

- Chinese culture values silence, "and women experiencing the pain of childbirth typically believe they will dishonor themselves and their families by a loud or wild response to pain" (Weber, 1996).

- Japanese Americans regard pain as an integral part of illness and traditionally exhibit a stoic attitude toward it. Some Japanese Americans feel that it is disgraceful to express pain verbally, even when their perception of the pain is intense. Patients may refuse pain medication when offered. Gordon (1997) reported that the Japanese tend to hide their pain under a stoic or unemotional demeanor. They may not readily "admit to being in pain and probably will not want to be touched as a comfort measure."

- Filipino Americans tend to view pain as "God's will for my life" and believe that neither the patient nor the physician should interfere with God's plan. Some Filipinos believe that illness may be attributed to a punishment from God and it would not be appropriate to interfere. Refusal of pain medication may be grounded in deep religious beliefs and should be respected. Some Filipino patients, especially the elderly, tend to hide their pain (Gordon, 1997; Kumasaka, 1996).

Black Americans form the largest minority cultural group in the United States. Recall from Chapter 2 that black American culture consists of several highly diverse subcultural groups. Depending on their cultural background, some black patients may deny or avoid dealing with pain until it is unbearable and then seek emergency care. Other blacks, who share mainstream attitudes about pain, may exhibit a stoic response to pain out of a desire to be a *perfect patient.* Still other black patients may feel that an overt reaction to pain poses a threat to their self-esteem and that denying the pain will be more acceptable to their caregivers. Black Americans with strong religious beliefs may believe that life on the earth (with all of its pain and suffering) is bearable only because there will be happiness and lack of pain after death.

White, Anglo-Saxon, American culture, currently the dominant cultural influence in the United States, comprises many diverse subcultural groups from many countries. White Anglo-Americans generally regard pain as a symptom of illness or injury. Evidence suggests that whites exhibit a moderate level of pain tolerance, express pain behavior more readily than blacks, and are more likely to seek pain relief. The majority of whites seek professional attention when their symptoms interfere with their vocation or avocational activity.

Native Americans are from an estimated 300 Indian nations; they reside mostly in the western part of the United States. Each Native American community has its own distinctive characteristic style of dealing with pain. However, in general, Native Americans are quiet in voice and demeanor, and they traditionally exhibit a stoic attitude and tolerate a high level of pain (Weber, 1996). Some patients may not seek pain relief and may tolerate pain until they are physically disabled.

Pain: Using Transcultural Communication to Plan Care

When patients are from other cultures, plan to use transcultural communication to assess pain, plan care, intervene with pain control measures, teach patients about pain interventions, and provide information about pain control. It is also important to talk with patients about their view of pain, previous pain control practices, knowledge regarding the source or cause of the pain, and preferences and expectations regarding pain relief. In addition, you should examine your own beliefs and values regarding pain and demonstrate the importance you place on pain control by responding quickly and appropriately to relieve the patient's pain.

Pain assessment, care planning, and intervention are parts of an ongoing process. Reassessments and evaluation should also be continuous and ongoing. It is important to thoroughly assess and document the patient's physiologic reactions, verbal reports, and behavioral expressions of pain on a frequent basis.

> **•••• COMMUNICATION CONSIDERATIONS ••••**
>
> Remember that what the patient says about the pain is the single most reliable indicator of the nature and intensity of the pain (U.S. Department of Health and Human Services Public Health Services, 1992).

Two general goals for pain management are to (1) eliminate or reduce the severity of the pain and (2) enhance patient comfort and satisfaction. An interdisciplinary health care team should plan specific pain control measures that include the patient and family, when appropriate.

Both pharmacologic and nonpharmacologic therapies are used to control pain. You should evaluate the effects of drug and nondrug therapy on a frequent basis. You also need to encourage the patient to let you know when pain is relieved or not relieved by specific therapies. Pain control therapy can then be readjusted on the basis of what the patient says about the pain and pain relief.

> **• • • • COMMUNICATION CONSIDERATIONS • • • •**
>
> When language is a barrier, arrange for an interpreter to assist in obtaining information about the patient's pain and in interpreting pain control strategies for the patient.

Patients also need to learn about how to use nonpharmacologic pain control strategies. These strategies provide the patient with self-control measures that may be used alone or in conjunction with pharmacologic measures to enhance pain relief. Teaching patients nonpharmacologic pain control measures will enhance their sense of control over the pain.

Some examples of nonpharmacologic pain strategies are (U.S. Department of Health and Human Services Public Health Services, 1992):

Cognitive-Behavioral	Physical Agents
• Education and instruction	• Heat or cold applications
• Relaxation	• Massage, exercise, immobilization
• Imagery	• Transcutaneous electrical nerve
• Music distraction	stimulation
• Biofeedback	

Melzack and Wall's (1965) *gate control theory of pain* provides the theoretical explanation for pain and for the effectiveness of various pain control measures. The gate control theory suggests that a neural system composed of a specialized body of cells in the dorsal horn of the spinal cord acts as a gating mechanism that blocks or decreases the transmission of pain stimuli to the higher brain centers. In addition, sensory stimuli from the higher brain centers (e.g., auditory and visual centers) and selective brain processes, such as emotions and cognition, are able to transmit impulses that close the gate to incoming pain stimuli (Melzack & Wall, 1965; Walker, Tan, & George, 1995).

The *chemical pain control theory* suggests that the body manufactures endogenous substances or endorphins that have analgesic properties. These endorphins act by binding to opioid receptors in the brain and spinal cord and blocking the transmission of pain impulses.

Pain: Using Transcultural Communication to Explain, Counsel, and Console

Using transcultural communication is critically important when assessing, querying, teaching, and counseling patients from diverse cultures who are experiencing pain. To involve the patient and family in setting goals and planning pain control strategies that are culturally acceptable, you can:

- Communicate openness, acceptance, and a willingness to listen to their views about pain and its control.

- Respect patients' autonomy by accepting choices they make about pain control. Allow mentally competent patients to retain some sense of control over their lives, including pain control.

- Be available to the patient who is experiencing pain. Sitting with the patient may decrease the person's anxiety level as well as pain level.

- Provide information about pain control in a clear manner, repeating important information.

- Provide information graphically to help reduce any language problem. For example, use a line drawing of the body when discussing specific areas of pain or discomfort, and use a numerical scale when discussing or evaluating pain intensity. Patients may require many teaching sessions to learn how to adequately care for themselves or family members.

- Secure a clergy member or traditional healer for the patient if requested. Different ethnic and cultural groups derive solace and comfort from different spiritual sources.

- Listen to your patients' descriptions of their pain and the degree of pain relief.

- Seek the support of colleagues and health team members to assist you in exploring culture-specific pain management strategies.

USING TRANSCULTURAL COMMUNICATION TO ASSIST PATIENTS WHO ARE DYING

Death is an inevitable phenomenon that influences how one looks at life. Death also makes life seem more meaningful and poignant. It is the underlying reason that people aspire and strive to find meaning in life. Because death is universal, each culture has developed its own beliefs, mores, norms, standards, and restrictions regarding responses to dying and death. The meaning ascribed to illness and the actual language used to discuss illness and death are different in every culture.

The Death Phenomenon

Each society's teleological view of life influences its responses to the **death phenomenon**. Three general patterns of responses have been identified: *death-accepting*, *death-defying*, and *death-denying* (Rando, 1984).

1. **Death-accepting** is a common response in some primitive societies, such as the Fiji Islanders and Trobrianders. In these societies, death is viewed as inevitable and a natural part of the life cycle. Dying is one of the activities of daily living.

2. **Death-defying**, an earlier practice, was a common response in societies such as early Egypt.

3. **Death-denying** is an accepted response in the United States. Many Americans refuse to confront death and try to protect themselves from the realities of death. Death is viewed as antithetical to living and not a normal part of human existence.

Transcultural Differences in Responses to Dying

Mexican Americans consider death as God's will. Mexican Americans' concept of death and an afterlife is deeply rooted in Roman Catholicism. They generally believe that enduring sickness is a sign of strength. When a patient is terminally ill, the family is involved in all aspects of decision making.

Asian Americans have different views about death depending on their particular subculture.

• *Chinese* culture holds bipolar views regarding death. One view is that death is only the vanishing of the human body; the true body exists forever. They believe that nature should be allowed to take its course, especially when a patient is suffering. Chinese philosophy has long advocated the right to choose death. The second view is that life should be valued and preserved at all costs and that health care providers should do all within their power to save lives, even when the patient is suffering from a painful and incurable disease (Corr, Nabe, & Corr, 1994).

- *Filipino Americans* tend to believe that people die because they have offended God or they are possessed by a spirit. They believe that dying is God's plan and that neither the patient nor the physician should interfere with God's will (Kumasaka, 1996).

- *Korean Americans'* traditional values dictate that patients should die at home.

Black Americans hold two belief systems regarding death (Jackson, 1980). The first belief system (based on the sacred norm) suggests that death provides an escape from this world and that people should look for glory in the afterworld. The second belief system (based on the secular norm) suggests that death is part of the normal life process and an inevitable event. Death should also be accepted as a constant companion. The secular norm assumes that death is a natural event, despite its highly disturbing social and emotional impact (Corr et al., 1994).

In many spirituals and in poetry written by black authors, the following themes are common: death as *freedom, rest, departure, finding peace, finding rest through closeness with Jesus,* and *a reward* (Corr et al., 1994).

White Anglo-Americans exhibit a wide array of emotions in response to the death of loved ones. Many respond to death with expressions of stoicism and a brave face rather than open expressions of grief. Spiritual beliefs and traditions vary among the subgroups. Many believe in immortality and place high value on family closeness (Pickett, 1993).

Native Americans view death as part of the life cycle: the old must die, and the young may die. Although most conceive of life and death as circular, Native American cultures deal with death in different ways. For instance, burial practices vary among tribal groups. Many tribal groups hold long, somber wakes at which food and memorial gifts are distributed. Some tribal groups mandate burying the deceased within 24 hours. Others forbid leaving the deceased alone and stipulate that a family member remain in attendance until the burial (Corr et al., 1994; Lawson, 1990).

Navajos fear death, and they distance themselves from death. Thus, Navajo patients often die in a hospital rather than at home. Navajos believe that patients with a terminal illness should be told that they may die. However, it is generally not acceptable to discuss death at length. Navajos respond to death and dying in a stoic manner. They are generally quiet in voice and demeanor. Navajos usually avoid touching the dead or dying person as well as items associated with death. Some Navajo nurses may have a healing ceremony performed after contact with a dead person.

COMMUNICATION CONSIDERATIONS

The Navajo language does not always have words that are similar in meaning to English words. To communicate with Navajo-speaking patients and families, use interpreters who are fluent in the Navajo language.

The *Luguna Pueblos* perform a prescribed ritual for burying the dead. The death ritual may be in the form of chanting or monotonous singing over the dead to frighten away evil spirits. They do not permit the body to be taken to a mortuary but perform the wrapping of the body themselves.

Dying: Using Transcultural Communication to Plan Care

Assisting patients to achieve an appropriate death requires effective transcultural communication and collaboration among patients, family members, and health care professionals. An **appropriate death** has been defined as a death one might choose, given the choice (Pickett, 1993). The essential components of an appropriate death are symptom control, comfort, and support. Showing respect for patients and family members and encouraging their active participation in decisions related to the patient's final days should guide your plan of care.

To help people from different cultures express their loss and grief in ways that are valued in their culture, you need to first clarify your own values and feelings about death, loss, and grief. Nurses who are consciously aware of their own values and preferences will be less likely to practice *cultural imposition*, which is the tendency to impose ones beliefs, values, and patterns of behavior upon patients from other cultures.

COMMUNICATION CONSIDERATIONS

It is critical that nurses recognize, understand, and respect each patient's and family's culture-specific values regarding dying and death.

Different cultures have different needs when confronted with dying and death. *Mexican Americans* view the nuclear and extended family as vitally important. The immediate and extended family is a primary source of social support, tangible aid, information, and advice, therefore, directing services toward the entire family is absolutely essential. Close friends are also primary sources of social support. It is important to provide family and friends with tangible aid, information, and advice.

Traditionally, the father or husband is the head of the Mexican household and may make all major decisions regarding the dying loved one. Mexican Americans who are separated from family and other contacts may feel a sense of isolation when faced with a dying child or relative, and consequently they are more likely to need the support of health team members.

Mexican Americans consider death to be God's will, a belief that is rooted in their religious heritage. They are very expressive in emotions and behavior. Mexican Americans may wish to have a priest present to perform last rites when a person is dying (Corr et al., 1994). Kind words and a gentle touch from the nurse convey a sense of caring, which will help to comfort the dying patient.

Asian Americans are very family oriented. The extended family should be involved in the care of the dying patient, because family members provide social support, resources, and tangible aid. Remember to incorporate relevant cultural values when planning care for the dying patient who is Asian. For example, Asian Americans have a deep respect for the body. Asians may feel that the body is not their own possession but is passed down from their ancestors. Some Asians believe that the head is sacred, and they consider it disrespectful to touch the head without permission. They may also consider it disrespectful to make direct eye contact.

When planning care for the dying patient, care providers must remember that many Asian and Islamic women are afraid of being examined by a male. They prefer being examined by a female whenever possible. When they are examined by a male, the unnecessary removal of underclothing should be avoided, and a female should be in attendance.

• • • COMMUNICATION CONSIDERATIONS • • •

When communicating and interacting with the dying patient's family, remember that smiling and nodding do not necessarily reflect understanding or agreement. Actually, for many Asians, smiling and nodding are signs of respect.

Many Asians feel that a sick person should never be left alone. This need may be accommodated by allowing family members to remain with the dying patient at all times.

Black Americans are also family oriented, and the extended family is very important. It is customary for many family members to remain with a dying patient in the hospital. Although the family is central, friends and church members also provide support and comfort as they visit often and pray for the patient (Corr et al., 1994). Expressions of grief for the dying patient may include crying, screaming, and various other emotions and behaviors. Health care providers should involve the patient and family when planning and implementing care.

White Anglo-Americans, as members of a death-denying culture, may try to cheat death by using extraordinary measures to save lives, even when patients are clearly suffering and dying. The strong need by some nursing and medical personnel to prolong life at any cost is an example of a death-denying attitude. Even when death comes after a long and difficult illness, it seems to be the *American way* to restrain expressions of grief and face the death of loved ones with quiet stoicism. Most white Americans do value their families, and family closeness does provide a source of support when a family member is dying. Because middle-class Americans also value self-determination, it is important to involve the dying patient and the family in all aspects of decision making and care planning.

Native Americans view the family, both nuclear and extended, as being highly important. Being there for a dying family member is of prime importance. Ross (1981) reports that "many Native-Americans believe that the spirit of a dying person cannot leave the body until the family is there." It is not unusual for many members of the extended family to remain with the dying patient, in close proximity, until death has occurred (Lawson, 1990). For instance, restrictive hospital rules have no meaning for Navajo people, and they may resist leaving the dying patient's bedside just because "Visiting hours are over."

When you are planning care for the dying Native American patient, it is best to obtain information by listening to rather than by directly interviewing family members. Some Native Americans feel that talking about their dying loved one detracts from the spiritual context and may bring bad luck. In addition, Native Americans may refuse to answer questions because they are suspicious of people of European descent. However, you may be able to overcome the family's initial reluctance to talk with you by showing respect and being sensitive to their point of view (Lawson, 1990).

Dying: Using Transcultural Communication to Explain, Counsel, and Console

There are several important ways to help patients and families cope with the process of dying.

1. Help the family identify resources within their church or community to which they can turn for comfort and solace.

2. Recognize that members of different cultures need different types of support from their health care providers. Explain to the patient and family what types of help the hospital and community can provide.

3. Demonstrate a willingness to listen to the patient's and family's fears and concerns. Help the patient and family identify inner strengths or religious beliefs that will allow them to emotionally cope with the trauma of facing death.

4. Recognize that the family system is very important in most cultural groups. Always consider the family as a unit when planning care for a loved one who is dying. Evaluate how the family structure influences the patient's response to dying, as well as the family's role in providing solace and support. Facilitate transcultural communication by showing your respect for family members and including them in your plan of care.

5. Serve as an advocate for the patient and family by supporting cultural values that are important to them. For instance, allow patients to use traditional practices, including healers, if that is their wish.

USING TRANSCULTURAL COMMUNICATION TO ASSIST PEOPLE WHO ARE GRIEVING

Grief is a reaction that encompasses a broad range of feelings and behaviors that are associated with loss. It is a dynamic, pervasive process that occurs in phases, over time.

The Grieving Process

Expressions of grief vary from person to person, but they are almost always influenced by a person's ethnic and cultural background. *Thought patterns* that are commonly associated with the **grieving process** include:

- Disbelief
- Confusion
- Preoccupation
- Hallucinations

Behaviors that are frequently associated with the grieving process include:

- Sleep disturbances
- Appetite disturbances
- Absentminded behavior
- Social withdrawal
- Distressing dreams

- Restlessness

- Crying

- Treasuring objects of the loved one

Transcultural Differences in Response to Grief

Providing grief support to individuals and family members requires compassion, understanding, and acceptance of how cultural traditions influence the grieving process. *Mexican Americans* perceive death to be God's will, and the culture dictates open expressions of grief. Religious practices such as praying for the dead and saying the rosary are significant aspects of the grieving process. The family is a source of support. Family members will need time and a private room where they can openly express their grief.

Asian Americans encompass many diverse cultural groups, with many different grieving patterns. Chinese are not publicly expressive of grief; however, some Chinese will feel comfortable venting their feelings, even when in public. Religious traditions are particularly important during stressful times. Japanese Americans respond to grief with denial or repression of emotions, which is an integral part of their culture. Because disclosure of feelings is viewed as bad manners, Japanese people are likely to be stoic when grieving (Corr et al., 1994; Pickett, 1993).

Black Americans may express their grief by crying and sometimes by screaming, praying, singing, and reading scriptures. The family, minister, and friends are major sources of support. Black Americans should be allowed the time and a private area where they can express their grief (Corr et al., 1994).

White Anglo-Americans typically respond to grief with stoiscism and restrained emotions. However, expressions of sadness and the demonstration of emotions vary among white Americans. Family closeness and their religious traditions are significant sources of support (Ross, 1981).

Native Americans may or may not express grief publicly. However, they may fully express their emotions if they are in a sympathetic environment. Grief tends to be family oriented, with all members assuming roles in the grieving process.

Grief: Using Transcultural Communication to Plan Care

Cultural assessment provides the basis for planning culturally specific care for grieving family members. Transcultural communication helps to facilitate assessment and collaborative planning as well as the development and refinement of intervention strategies that can be used to support grieving families. The cultural assessment should include data such as the family's ethnic or racial identity, value orientation, language or dialect, and family structure. These data can be used to plan culturally specific care.

COMMUNICATION CONSIDERATIONS

As you perform your assessment and plan care, use an unhurried approach to show respect, compassion, and sensitivity for grieving family members.

Grief: Using Transcultural Communication to Explain, Counsel, and Console

You can help family members with the grieving process by following these steps.

1. Assist family members in dealing with their loss. Encourage each person to talk about the loss. Be a patient and active listener.

COMMUNICATION CONSIDERATIONS

Working with grieving families whose native language is not English will require an interpreter, not only for exchanging information but also for understanding finer shades of meaning.

2. Assist the person in identifying and expressing feelings such as anger, anxiety, guilt, and helplessness. Family members may not want to discuss certain feelings because they are upsetting and unpleasant. Feelings that are left unexpressed may go unresolved for long periods of time or even permanently.

3. Provide the family with time to grieve. Allow the family to start coming to terms with their loss and all of its ramifications. Remind the family that grieving is a process that occurs in phases, over time. Sometimes, grieving family members and friends are eager to get over the loss and its pain and move back into a normal routine before they are ready.

4. Recognize that some points in time may be more difficult for the bereaved than others, such as the first anniversary of the death or certain holidays. One effective intervention is to help the person anticipate this problem and prepare for it.

5. Allow for individual as well as cultural differences. There is a wide range of behavioral responses to grief. Do not expect all family members who are grieving to grieve in the same way.

6. Help the person examine his or her defenses and coping styles. Some of the defenses and coping styles portend competent behaviors; others do not. For example, a person who copes by using alcohol or drugs excessively is probably not making an effective adjustment to the loss. This person should be helped to explore other coping strategies.

7. Provide continuing support as necessary. Some people require continuing support over a long period of time. One way to offer continuing support is through support groups. There are special groups for persons who have lost a spouse, children, parents, and other loved ones. There are also groups within each culture that offer help and comfort to the bereaved. It is important to be aware of community and cultural resources and to make referrals, when necessary.

REFERENCES

Corr, C. A., Nabe, C. M., & Corr, D. M. (1994). *Death and dying, life and living* (pp. 73–121). Pacific Grove, CA.: Brooks/Cole.

Gordon, C. (1997). The effect of cancer pain on quality of life in different ethnic groups: A literature review. *Nurse Practitioner Forum, 3*(1), 5–13.

Hughes, O. M. (1997). Caring for people in pain. In J. Luckmann (Ed.), *Saunder's manual of nursing care.* Philadelphia: Saunders.

Jackson, M. (1980). The black experience with death: A brief analysis through black writings. In R. A. Kalish (Ed.), *Death and dying: Views from many cultures* (pp. 92–97). New York: Baywood.

Klessig, J. (1992). Cross-cultural medicine—A decade later. *Western Journal of Medicine, 157* [Special issue], 316–322.

Kumasaka, L. (1996). 'My pain is God's will.' *American Journal of Nursing, 96*(6), 45–47.

Lawson, L. V. (1990). Culturally sensitive support for grieving parents. *American Journal of Maternal/Child Nursing, 15*(2), 76–79.

Ludwig-Beymer, P. (1995). Transcultural aspects of pain. In M. M. Andrews & J. S. Boyle, *Transcultural concepts in nursing care.* Philadelphia: Lippincott.

Melzack, R., & Wall, P. D. (1965). Pain mechanism: A new theory. *Science, 150*(36), 971–972.

Pickett, M. (1993). Cultural awareness in the context of terminal illness. *Cancer Nursing, 16*(2), 102–106.

Rando, T. A. (1984). *Grief, dying, and death.* Champaign, IL.: Research Press.

Ross, H. M. (1981). Societal/cultural views regarding death and dying. *Topics in Clinical Nursing, 174,* 1–13.

Salerno, E. (1995). Race, culture, and medications. *Journal of Emergency Nursing, 21*(6), 560–562.

U.S. Department of Health and Human Services Public Health Services. (1992, February). *Acute pain management: Clinical practice guidelines.* AHCPR Pub. No. 92-0032. Rockville, MD: Agency for Health Care Policy and Research.

Villarruel, A. M., & Ortiz de Montellano, B. (1992). Culture and pain: A mesoamerican perspective. *Advanced Nursing Science, 15*(1), 21–32.

Walker, A. C., Tan, L., & George, S. (1995). Impact of culture on pain management: An Australian nursing perspective. *Holistic Nursing Practice, 9*(2), 48–57.

Weber, S. E. (1996). Cultural aspects of pain in childbearing women. *Journal of Obstetric, Gynecologic, and Neonatal Nursing, 25*(1), 67–72.

Zatzick, D. F., & Dimsdale, J. (1990). Cultural variations in response to painful stimuli. *Psychosomatic Medicine, 52*(5), 544–557.

SUGGESTED READINGS

Banks, L. J. (1992). Counseling. In G. M. Bulechek & J. C. McCloskey (Eds.), *Nursing intervention* (2nd ed.). Philadelphia: Elsevier.

Battaglia, B. (1998). Cultural views on death and dying: Part 3. *Cross-Cultural Connection, 3*(3), 1–4.

Braun, K., Pietsch, J., & Blanchette, P. (2000). *Cultural issues in end-of-life decision-making.* London: Sage Publication.

Cowles, K. V. (1996). Cultural perspectives of grief: An expanded concept analysis. *Journal of Advanced Nursing, 23,* 287–294.

Doorenbos, A., & Nies, M., (2003). The use of advance directives in a population of Asian Indian Hindus. *Journal of Transcultural Nursing, 14*(1), 17–24.

Duggleby, W. (2002). The language of pain at the end of life. *Pain Management Nursing, 3*(4), 154–160.

Eng, J. L. (1998, October 18). Health workers trying to bridge cultural gaps: Study explores ethnic differences in approaching death and dying. *Seattle Times*, p. B8.

Geissler, E. M. (1998). *Cultural assessment.* St. Louis: Mosby.

Giger, J. N., & Davidhizar, R. E. (1995). *Transcultural nursing, assessment and interventions.* St. Louis: Mosby.

Leininger, M. (1995). *Transcultural nursing: Concepts, theories, research and practices.* New York: McGraw-Hill.

Leininger, M. (1997). Understanding cultural pain for improved health care. *Journal of Transcultural Nursing, 9*(1), 32–35.

Muñoz, C. (2001, March). Cultural concepts to consider in the care of the ethnically diverse client and family. *Ohio Nurses Review,* 12–18.

Nishimoto, P., & Foley, J. (2001). Cultural beliefs of Asian Americans associated with terminal illness and death. *Seminars in Oncology Nursing, 17*(3), 179–189.

Nyatanga, B. (2002). Culture, palliative care and multiculturalism. *International Journal of Palliative Nursing, 8*(5), 240–246.

Payne, R. (2002). Viewpoints, improving palliative care for African American and other minority patients. *Oncology Times, 24*(5), 2.

Perry, H. L. (1993). Mourning and funeral customs of African Americans. In B. O. Irish, J. E. Jenkins, & B. L. Lundquist (Eds.), *Ethnic variations in dying, death, and grief: Diversity in universality.* Washington, DC: Taylor & Francis.

Salimbene, J. (2000). *What language does your patient hurt in?* Amherst, MA: Diversity Resources Publication.

Younoszai, B. (1993). Mexican American perspectives related to death. In B. O. Irish, J. E. Jenkins, & B. L. Lundquist (Eds.), *Ethnic variations in dying, death, and grief: Diversity in universality* (pp. 67–99). Washington, DC: Taylor & Francis.

UNIT FOUR
EVALUATION

EVALUATING YOUR TRANSCULTURAL COMMUNICATION SKILLS IN PLANNING AND IMPLEMENTING CARE

The following exercises highlight some of the concepts that we discussed in this unit. Make a note if you are selecting a different option than you would have before studying Chapters 13 and 14.

Exercise One: Evaluating How Comfortable You Feel When Planning and Implementing Care for Patients from Diverse Cultures

Recall that you performed this exercise before you began your study of this unit. By now you should have read Chapters 13 and 14. You may also have had some new experiences in planning care, patient teaching, providing pain relief, and assisting dying patients and grieving relatives.

The following statements contain assignments that you may have received as you cared for patients from diverse cultures. Using the following five levels of comfort, rate how comfortable you *now* feel about performing each assignment. Compare your current levels of comfort with your earlier levels.

- Level 1: I feel very uncomfortable.
- Level 2: I feel rather uncomfortable.
- Level 3: I feel fairly comfortable.
- Level 4: I feel comfortable.
- Level 5: I feel very comfortable.

1. *Assignment:* Talk with a patient about his financial and home situation—two factors that can influence your plan of care.   **1 2 3 4 5**

2. *Assignment:* Explain to a Japanese patient who regularly uses soy sauce and other similar flavorings that he must reduce the sodium in his diet to control his congestive heart failure.   **1 2 3 4 5**

3. *Assignment:* Negotiate a biomedical plan of care with a patient from a culture that does not totally accept biomedical practices.

   1 2 3 4 5

4. *Assignment:* Witness a patient's signing of an *Informed Consent* before a major procedure. **1 2 3 4 5**

5. *Assignment:* Develop clear, realistic, and measurable learning objectives for a patient who needs to learn about his medications, diet, rest, and activity schedule before going home. **1 2 3 4 5**

6. *Assignment:* Teach a patient a procedure such as changing a dressing or self-administration of insulin. **1 2 3 4 5**

7. *Assignment:* Work closely with an interpreter to teach a patient with limited English proficiency about his diet and medications.

1 2 3 4 5

8. *Assignment:* Counsel a patient with chronic pain who is from an emotive culture: for example, the Italian culture. **1 2 3 4 5**

9. *Assignment:* Counsel and console a dying patient and his family who are observing cultural and religious rituals with which you are unfamiliar.

1 2 3 4 5

Exercise Two: Evaluating Your Point of View toward Transcultural Nursing Situations That Involve Planning, Teaching, Counseling, and Consoling

You performed this exercise earlier in the self-assessment section of this unit. Select the answers that best describe your point of view *now* that you have completed the chapters in this unit. There is no scoring for these questions.

1. When planning care for patients from diverse cultures, you should
   a. make every effort to preserve the patients' cultural practices
   b. consider the patients' cultural practices, but make the biomedical aspects of the patients' care plan your major priority
   c. convince the patients that they should follow the medical and nursing care plan for their own good
   d. let the patients manage their own care as much as possible

2. A patient who refuses to follow a biomedical plan of care
   a. needs to have logical reasons for his refusal to follow the plan
   b. is being unreasonable and noncompliant
   c. Is observing his legal and constitutional rights
   d. Is recklessly endangering his health and should be scheduled for a psychiatric consult

3. When teaching patients from diverse cultures
   a. I try to provide the same information in the same way, regardless of a patient's cultural background.
   b. I try to consider each patient's special learning needs and limitations that are related to his or her culture or lack of proficiency in English.
   c. I don't believe that is possible to write measurable learning objectives for patients.
   d. I realize that sometimes it is necessary to negotiate with patients and adapt my teaching plan to their cultural views and daily patterns.

4. When caring for patients from diverse cultures who are experiencing pain
   a. I realize that some patients are stoic in their response to pain, whereas other patients are emotive.
   b. It is difficult to evaluate a patient's pain when the person responds in a stoic manner and refuses to acknowledge that the pain exists.
   c. It is difficult to work with patients who scream and cry when in pain.
   d. The patient's own description of his or her pain is often inaccurate.

5. When caring for patients from diverse cultures who are dying
   a. I try to accept each patient's cultural values and behavior patterns regarding dying and death.
   b. I find it difficult to deal with the dying patient's family when their continuous presence makes it hard for me to provide care.
   c. I don't know what to say when family members express their grief to me after the patient's death.
   d. I don't feel that I have the experience to counsel a bereaved family from another culture.

Exercise Three: Reviewing Your *Transcultural Interaction Diary*

1. Have you had an opportunity to write a nursing care plan or a teaching plan for a patient from another culture? _____

2. How did your patient react to your plan? Did the person find the plan acceptable, partially acceptable, or unacceptable because of his or her cultural beliefs? _____

3. If partially acceptable or unacceptable, what did you do or say to negotiate with the patient? _____

Were you able to reach a satisfactory compromise with the patient?

_____

If you were unable to reach a compromise, were you able to accept the patient's decisions regarding his or her own care and learning needs?

_____

4. What teaching methods have you been using when instructing patients about their care? _____

_____

Which method do you feel most comfortable with? _____

Have you been able to follow a patient's progress after discharge?

_____

Has the patient continued to follow your instructions?

_____

5. How do you plan to improve your teaching plans and activities?

_____

_____

6. Have you had an opportunity to assess patients from other cultures who responded stoically to pain? _____

What did you do to assess the patient?

_____

_____

What did you do to relieve the patient's pain?

_____

_____

7. Have you had an opportunity to assess patients from other cultures who responded emotionally to pain? _____

What communication techniques did you use to assess the patient?

_____

_____

What did you do to relieve the patient's pain?

_____

_____

8. Have you been assigned a patient from another culture who is dying?

_____

What religious and cultural practices did the patient and family observe?

_____

_____

How did you feel about these practices? Comfortable or uncomfortable?

_____

9. What did you say and do to comfort the patient? _____

_____

_____

What did you say and do to console the grieving family? _____

_____

_____

10. What can you do to improve your transcultural communication in situations that involve dying, death, and grieving?

_____

_____

Exercise Four: Evaluating Your Knowledge of Transcultural Communication Principles That Are Related to Planning and Implementing Care

Write a brief response to these questions, which are drawn from topics discussed in Chapters 13 and 14.

1. In general, developing a care plan involves four steps:
   a. _____
   b. _____
   c. _____
   d. _____

2. To meet American Nurses Association standards, a care plan must be:
   a. _____
   b. _____
   c. _____
   d. _____
   e. _____

3. Leininger recommends the following three approaches when planning care for patients from diverse cultures:

    a. _____

    b. _____

    c. _____

4. The Patient Self-Determination Act (PSDA) guarantees patients the right to: _____

    _____

5. The five steps of the teaching/learning process are:

    a. _____

    b. _____

    c. _____

    d. _____

    e. _____

6. The nursing diagnosis *knowledge deficit* is used inaccurately because:

    _____

    _____

7. Learning styles vary for patients from diverse cultures. Four types of learning styles are:

    a. _____

    b. _____

    c. _____

    d. _____

8. The five major steps of the *LEARN model* developed by Berlin and Fowkes are:

    a. _____

    b. _____

    c. _____

    d. _____

9. Five steps that are involved in teaching procedures to patients from diverse cultures are:

    a. _____

    b. _____

    c. _____

    d. _____

    e. _____

10. Pain is defined as: _____

_____

11. Members of different cultural groups tend to respond to pain in different ways. Mexican Americans tend to view pain as: _____

_____

Asian Americans tend to view pain as: _____

_____

Black Americans tend to view pain as: _____

_____

White Anglo-Saxon Americans tend to view pain as: _____

_____

Native Americans tend to view pain as:

_____

12. Describe six ways to use transcultural communication to plan care for patients who are in pain:
    a. _____
    b. _____
    c. _____
    d. _____
    e. _____
    f. _____

13. Three general patterns of responses to death are:
    a. _____
    b. _____
    c. _____

14. Describe five ways you can use transcultural communication to advise, counsel, and console people from diverse cultures who are going through the death experience:
    a. _____
    b. _____
    c. _____
    d. _____
    e. _____

15. Thought patterns associated with the grieving process include:

_____

_____

16. Behaviors associated with the grieving process include:

_____

_____

17. Describe seven ways you can use transcultural communication to advise, counsel, and console people from diverse cultures who are grieving:

    a. _____

    b. _____

    c. _____

    d. _____

    e. _____

    f. _____

    g. _____

UNIT FIVE

Transcultural Communication Skills between Health Care Providers

UNIT FIVE ASSESSMENT

ASSESSING YOUR TRANSCULTURAL COMMUNICATION SKILLS WITH OTHER HEALTH CARE PROVIDERS

Exercise One: Assessing Your Personal Objectives

Until now, you have primarily studied how to communicate with patients from other cultures. This unit discusses barriers to transcultural communication between health care providers and presents techniques for overcoming those barriers.

What do you want to gain from studying this unit? Check those points in the following list that apply to you and write down any other objectives.

My personal objectives are to:

_____ Learn how to relate better to staff members or nursing students who are from other cultures.

_____ Identify and overcome biases and prejudices that are hindering me from working successfully with nurses from other cultures.

_____ Sharpen my skills in supervising ancillary personnel from diverse cultures.

_____ Decrease the frustration I feel when working with physicians or nurses who are not proficient in English or who have a strong accent.

_____ Welcome working with skilled foreign nurses and appreciate the wealth of knowledge concerning other cultures that I can gain from them.

_____ Learn more about how to manage a diverse nursing staff.

_____ Learn about how conflicts are resolved in the workplace.

My other personal objectives for learning how to communicate in a diverse workplace are to:

1. _____

2. _____

3. _____

4. _____

5. _____

306

Exercise Two: Assessing Your Personal Responses to Working with Care Providers from Different Cultures

In today's diverse workplace, you will need to work closely with registered nurses, nursing students, physicians, and ancillary personnel who are from different cultures and who speak English as a second language. How do you *really feel* about working with providers who are from foreign countries, or from different racial or ethnic groups? Take a minute to answer the following questions. You do not need to share your answers with anyone, so be honest with yourself.

	Agree	Neutral	Disagree
I would rather work with an American nurse than a foreign nurse.	_____	_____	_____
I find it frustrating to work with nurses or physicians who are not proficient in English.	_____	_____	_____
If I thought that a nurse or physician was not fulfilling duties because of cultural or language problems, I would hesitate to report the person for fear that I would be considered prejudiced.	_____	_____	_____
I enjoy working with a skilled foreign nurse. I feel that I can learn a lot from this person.	_____	_____	_____
I like to attend classes and informal meetings where I can learn more about how nurses from other countries are educated.	_____	_____	_____
I do not feel prepared to work with or supervise an unlicensed assistive worker who has some problems with understanding English.	_____	_____	_____

Exercise Three: Using Your *Transcultural Interaction Diary*

In Unit One, you set up and started your *Transcultural Interaction Diary*. Since then, you have been primarily recording your transcultural interactions with patient, families, and interpreters.

1. Today, set up a new section in your diary for recording significant trans-cultural interactions with supervising nurses, staff nurses, physicians, unlicensed assistive personnel, and other nursing students.

2. Start using your diary now, before reading this chapter. Try to remember and record any past interactions that were either very positive or very negative. For each interaction, write down both the verbal and nonverbal transcultural communications that passed between you and the other health care provider. Record the feelings and thoughts that you had during and after each interaction.

3. Continue to keep your diary as you study this chapter. Try to use the various suggestions from the chapter for improving your transcultural communication with health providers from different cultures. Note how using a particular technique helped to clarify your communications.

4. Remember to keep your diary in a private place. You will not feel as free to write about your positive and negative transcultural interactions with staff members if other people might read your personal experiences.

CHAPTER 15

Fostering Transcultural Communication with Other Health Care Providers

KEY TERMS

- Arbitration
- Collectivism
- Conflict Resolution
- External Locus of Control
- Individualism
- Internal Locus of Control
- Mediation
- Negotiation
- Perceived Injurious Experience
- Unperceived Injurious Experience

OBJECTIVES

After completing this chapter, you should be able to:

- Discuss the major barriers that impede transcultural communication between health care providers from different cultures.
- Distinguish between the values of individualism and collectivism in the workplace, and give an example of each.
- Identify at least 10 approaches that you can use to improve your transcultural communication with co-workers and ancillary personnel.
- Identify strategies that a nurse-manager can use to improve transcultural communication in the workplace.
- Discuss the dynamics of transcultural conflict in the workplace, and describe alternative methods for resolving workplace disputes.

INTRODUCTION

In addition to bridging the transcultural gap between themselves and their patients, nurses must learn how to communicate with medical personnel from around the globe. The nursing and medical workforce of today is dramatically different from the workforce of the past. National surveys reveal that enrollment in nursing schools continues to decline and that fewer people choose nursing as their career. As a result of this shortage in the nursing workforce, a lot of nurses become overburdened, overworked, and overstressed. Dissatisfaction in their job becomes inevitable. Although the solution to the nursing shortage needs to be multifaceted and comprehensive, recruitment of foreign graduates has become a common response to this issue. Since the mid-1990s, large urban hospitals (primarily on the East and West Coasts and in the Sun Belt) have recruited foreign nurses to meet staffing demands (Williams & Rodgers, 1993). Moreover, the work and economic conditions in this country have attracted foreign nurses, primarily from the Philippines, Great Britain, Ireland, and Canada. In addition, the demand for ancillary personnel has increased the number of foreign workers and ethnically diverse minorities in the health care workplace. Unlicensed ancillary workers are expected to be the fastest growing health care occupational group in the twenty-first century.

A multicultural health care workforce can have a positive effect on patient care. Health care workers from diverse backgrounds bring a variety of experiences and a wide range of knowledge to the health care setting. Nurses who are from different cultures offer fresh ideas and different solutions to long-term problems. Foreign nurses can help American nurses understand and relate better to patients who are also from diverse cultural backgrounds.

On the other hand, the cultural diversity of the workforce may raise barriers that can produce serious workplace problems. Foreign nurses are usually competent and committed workers; nevertheless, daily interactions with native English-speaking nurses and physicians can be strained. American nurses may feel that foreign nurses are not as technically proficient as nurses educated in the United States. Furthermore, some foreign nurses come to the United States with their own biases, and they may feel that American nurses lack competence and compassion. In addition, ancillary personnel from diverse backgrounds may misunderstand and resent the white American nurses who are in charge. Openness and respect of differences become crucial in maintaining good working relationships.

The major barriers to transcultural communication between staff members, the potential conflicts, and some possible solutions and resolutions are presented in the sections that follow.

BARRIERS TO TRANSCULTURAL COMMUNICATION BETWEEN HEALTH CARE PROVIDERS

Barriers to transcultural communication between health care providers extend from confused pronouns and foreign terminology to different values that result in different nursing styles. Major barriers are:

- Different cultural patterns and biases that affect the relationships between physicians, nurses, and ancillary personnel.
- Racism and prejudice that can undermine professional relationships.
- Clashes in values that arise between foreign nurses and nurses trained in the United States.
- Different perceptions of nursing responsibilities and patient care that are based on different cultural values.
- Differences in time orientation.
- Different systems of nursing and medical education.
- Language differences that result in serious miscommunications.

Other factors that may affect the attitudes and performance of health care providers from different cultures are (Lajkowicz, 1993):

1. The status of men, women, physicians, and nurses in the culture.
2. Attitudes toward authority figures.
3. Methods for financing health care.
4. Responsibilities of the patient's family for providing health care.
5. The use of artificial life-support systems.
6. The orientation to time as predominantly past oriented, present oriented, or future oriented.
7. The value of work as a health care provider.

Different Cultural Patterns and Biases

Cultural patterns and biases that staff members bring to the hospital can complicate communications and create misunderstandings and resentments. For example, many male physicians from the Middle East think of women as subservient. These physicians may feel that they have the right to shout at female nurses and demand assistance from them. American nurses, who have been raised to think of themselves as equal to men, may be upset by the physicians' tone of voice and condescending manner.

American nurses also can become frustrated by the lack of discussion, information sharing, and teamwork that often characterizes their relationships with physicians from the Middle East (Burner, Cunningham, & Hattar, 1990).

On the other hand, nurses from cultures that raise women to be subservient may find it difficult to be assertive when working with American nurses and physicians. For example, if a Japanese nurse does not agree with an order from a physician, she may follow the order without protest, providing the order is not harmful to the patient. In contrast, an American nurse who does not agree with the physician's order may challenge the order and argue with the physician. The Japanese nurse raised in the traditional Japanese culture may regard the American nurse as disrespectful of authority and guilty of causing the physician to "lose face."

Racism and Prejudice

Chapter 5 introduced the concept that racism exists in American nursing as a formidable barrier that severely undermines transcultural communication. According to Barbee (1993), there are certain attributes of nursing that prevent nurses from openly confronting the racism that exists in their profession. These attributes are:

- *An emphasis on empathy.* Nurses perceive themselves as caring individuals who see all people as the same rather than different. Nurses are taught that illness has no color and that their vocation is to help sick people, regardless of their color, creed, or race. This perception of themselves as caring makes it very difficult for nurses to acknowledge that they are capable of racism.

- *An individual orientation.* The major concepts that nurses learn in school are individualistic rather than group oriented. Although nursing theory seems to emphasize families, groups, and communities, nursing practice is geared to the needs of individuals. Also, schools of nursing require students to study the hard sciences such as chemistry and physics, whereas social sciences such as sociology and anthropology are usually electives. As a consequence, nurses fail to learn enough about cultural diversity and the multicultural milieu in which they will be working.

- *A preference for homogeneity and a need to avoid conflict.* According to Brink (1990), selection committees on nursing faculties prefer a homogeneous student body because it tends to be more efficient, nonchallenging, and nonthreatening than a heterogeneous one.

Such characteristics reduce conflict and promote solidarity within the nursing ranks.

These attributes have allowed the following three types of racism to flourish in American nursing (Barbee, 1993):

1. *Denial.* There are several ways by which nurses can deny racism. Nurses—black and white—may simply refuse to use the term *race* or *racism*. Black nurses may believe that their humanitarian work makes them immune to racism, and thus for them racism does not exist. White nurses may substitute the more benign terms of *ethnocentrism, cultural bias,* and *cultural diversity* for the politically incorrect term of *racism,* thereby denying its existence.

2. *Color-blind perspective.* Nurses who adhere to the color-blind perspective believe that race is a social category that has no relevance to an individual's behavior, and thus "individuals should not notice each other's racial group membership" (Barbee, 1993). For those who adopt the color-blind perspective, race is a taboo topic, and they view social relationships as interpersonal rather than intergroup relationships.

   The color-blind perspective helps nurses to (a) avoid overt conflict with people of other races, (b) minimize the discomfort and embarrassment that is associated with discussions of race and racism, (c) ignore or distort the fact that cultural differences exist, and (d) protect themselves from charges of discrimination in the workplace.

3. *Aversive racism.* According to Barbee (1993), "aversive racism is characterized by ambivalence: feelings and beliefs associated with an egalitarian value system conflict with unacknowledged negative feelings and beliefs concerning blacks." This form of racism is subtle because aversive racists do not see themselves as prejudiced or discriminatory in any way.

   Although racism distorts transcultural communication, prejudices between the nationalities, social classes, and sexes *within a culture* can also cause communication problems. For example, prejudices within the Hispanic culture may make professionals from the Dominican Republic reluctant to work with Puerto Ricans. Second-generation Mexican American nurses may not want to take orders from Central American nurses or physicians. Some black men object to working for black women. Some Latin men refuse to take directions from Latin or black women (Burner, 1990).

Different Value Systems

Different value systems can also complicate transcultural communication between staff members. Staff nurses from different cultures may have:

1. Different perceptions of staff responsibilities to each other.
2. Different perceptions of the nurse's role in patient care.
3. A different locus of control.

Different Perceptions of Staff Responsibilities. Recall from Chapter 2 that cultural values deeply influence what a person feels is most important: the welfare of the individual or the welfare of the group. **Individualism** emphasizes the importance of individual rights and rewards. **Collectivism** emphasizes the importance of group decisions and places the rights of the group as a whole above the rights of any individual in the group.

> **Example:** Unlike Western nurses, Asian nurses tend to accept difficult assignments without complaint. They also may be more willing to do what American nurses might consider demeaning (e.g., cleaning cabinets).
>
> Because many Asian nurses value *the group*, they believe that a nurse's individual duties have less value than the combined work of all of the nurses on the unit.

Also, when assigned to difficult or menial tasks, nurses from Asian cultures may feel it is inappropriate to confront a supervisor and demand a change of assignment. Maintaining face and ensuring harmony are Eastern cultural values that may be more important to Asian nurses than upsetting their supervisor in order to get an easier assignment. Indeed, an emphasis on minimizing conflict, maintaining harmony, teamwork, and commitment to group loyalty typify most Asian cultures.

In contrast, nurses educated in Western culture generally place more value on individualism and independence. Thus, Western nurses may complain to the supervisor if they feel assignments are unfair or involve menial work. This assertive behavior is consistent with ingrained values of equitable work distribution and the respect for education and professionalism that define the American work style.

Western nurses also want to be *individually* recognized for their work; for instance, they may want a promotion, or they may dream of being publicly honored for giving outstanding patient care or other accomplishments.

Different Perceptions of the Nurse's Role. Nurses from different cultures have different perceptions of the nurse's role and nursing care values, which American nurses may not appreciate.

Example: In a study of Philippine American nurses, the most important finding was the theme of *obligation to care* that prevailed in all aspects of their work (Spangler, 1992). This theme, which epitomized the Philippine American nurses' values, was expressed in three important ways:

1. *Expressed seriousness and dedication to work.* These nurses felt a strong sense of duty toward their patients, which was fully developed during their years in nursing school.

2. *Attentiveness to the patient's physical comfort needs.* In the words of one nurse:

   > To me, it is very important that patients are physically comfortable. I clean them up . . . . I talk to them while I attend to their physical needs. With our busy schedule, this is the best time to get to know the patients.

   In contrast, mainstream American nurses tended to devalue the physical care of patients because of its association with the body and body products. Indeed, some American nurses regarded the physical care of patients as menial work. According to one Philippine American nurse, "Here in the United States, the prestige is when you are away from the bedside; actual patient care is relegated to nurse's aides."

3. *Respect and patience.* The Philippine cultural values of respect and patience were learned early in life by the nurses and were carried forth into their relationships with patients. As expressed by a Philippine American nurse:

   > We are very patient people so I think that is reflected in our work. We tolerate demanding patients a bit more. Some Americans tell us, "How can you tolerate that patient? I would have told him off a long time ago."

In summary, the theme of an obligation to care reflected the Phillipine American nurses' strong belief that bedside nursing is truly the core of nursing. This value conflicted with the attitude of some American nurses that the physical care of patients is devalued work with low prestige and should therefore be delegated to ancillary personnel.

Differences in Locus of Control. *Locus of control* refers to the degree of control that individuals feel that they have over events. People who feel in control of their environment have an **internal locus of control**. People who believe that luck, fate, or chance controls their lives have an **external locus of control**.

Health care providers who are trained in the United States typically have an internal locus of control. American physicians and nurses feel that it is their duty to diagnose disorders, plan interventions, carry out procedures, and do everything possible to save the patient's life.

Conversely, health care providers from cultures that promote an external locus of control (some Mexican Americans, Appalachians, and Puerto Ricans) may have a more fatalistic attitude toward their patients and thus feel that they cannot control matters of life and death. For example, when a patient who is expected to die does die on the operating room table, care providers with an external locus of control may be puzzled when the hospital administration asks for a quality review of the case (Giger & Davidhizar, 1996).

Finally, the cultural beliefs of some American Indians, Chinese Americans, and Japanese Americans may not fall under the concept of locus of control. These cultural groups believe themselves to be in harmony with nature, rather than being controlled by nature or in control of nature (Giger & Davidhizar, 1996).

Differences in Time Orientation

Recall from Chapter 2 that cultural groups are either past, present, or future oriented. Americans generally value the future over the present. Southern blacks and Puerto Ricans value the present over the future. Southern Appalachians, traditional Chinese Americans, and Mexican Americans value the present.

The ways in which different cultural groups value time can create challenges in the health care workplace. For example, people who work in the operating room (OR) must be both future and present oriented. To plan and adhere to the OR schedule, the person must be future oriented and abide by the calendar and clock. However, once the surgical procedure begins, the surgeon and nurses must now switch to a present orientation (Giger & Davidhizar, 1996).

Staff meetings also are influenced by the time orientation of staff members. For instance, staff members who are meeting to plan for the future may become annoyed with members who want to spend all of the time on present-day problems and issues.

Educational Differences

The fact that foreign nurses are educated differently from American nurses raises yet another potential barrier to communication. Generally, nursing education outside of the United States is less theory oriented, focusing primarily on the development of clinical skills. Also, there is less emphasis on meeting the psychosocial needs of patients. As a result, foreign-educated nurses may be less inclined to use therapeutic touch with patients or to engage patients in conversations that build trust and rapport.

Also, because most non-Western cultures value emotional restraint, foreign-educated nurses may not be trained to intervene when patients are experiencing grief or loss. Moreover, nurses from non-Western cultures may feel that grief and loss are private family matters and that it is the family's responsibility to assist the patient (Burner, 1990).

Another cultural difference in the education of nurses revolves around *who* provides the majority of care—the nurse, the patient's family, or the patient. Recall that the Philippine American nurses felt it was the *nurse's duty* to give patients complete physical care. Other nurses, educated outside of the United States, may have been taught that it is the *family's duty* to bathe the patient and provide personal care. For example, in the Far East and in rural hospitals in Africa, a family member usually bathes the patient. As a result of this training, a foreign-born nurse may be reluctant to provide morning care to patients.

In contrast, nurses educated in the United States are taught that patients should perform *self-care* whenever possible. In keeping with the American values of independence and self-reliance, American nurses encourage patients to be ambulatory, active, and self-sufficient as soon as possible.

Even when nurses are from other English-speaking countries, they are educated differently from American nurses. English nurses, taught under the system of socialized medicine, may find it difficult to adjust to the concept that health care in the United States is a business, and physicians are in private practice. These nurses may not be familiar with physician referral services, charging patients for supplies, or the use of extreme measures to prolong the lives of terminally ill patients.

Language Differences

Language differences, perhaps more than any other barrier, raise the potential for serious miscommunications between health care providers. Today, large medical centers in the United States may be primarily staffed by nurses and physicians for whom English is a second language. For example, in urban medical centers on the East Coast, it is not unusual to hear a Filipino nurse and a Haitian nurse attempting to communicate with a resident physician who has been educated in India. Unless these caregivers take the time to clarify their communications, serious errors may result. Even when only the nurse is foreign born, the potential for miscommunication exists (especially over the telephone), unless words are clarified by a co-worker or physician.

> **Example:** A Filipino nurse who was temporarily assigned to an unfamiliar medical unit transcribed a telephone order from a physician. The physician said: "Give Johnson 50 ml of Demerol for pain. If she is still complaining of pain after an hour, call me and I'll increase the dosage." When transcribing the order, the nurse missed the physician's reference to the patient as *she*, a common error among Filipinos and some Chinese and Japanese speakers. *Mr.* Johnson, who happened to be on the same ward, might have received the medication had another nurse not questioned the order.

Language differences can also create communication problems between patients and nurses. Patients may feel apprehensive when they are assigned a foreign nurse (Burner, 1990). Patients may complain that foreign nurses do not understand what they are saying. For instance, the nurse may not comprehend the patient's request for a pain medication or assistance.

Furthermore, nonverbal communication can create misunderstandings. For example, an Asian nurse may think that it is rude to sustain prolonged eye contact with a patient; the patient, on the other hand, may interpret the lack of eye contact as lack of interest. As a result of this confusion, the patient may request an American nurse, a request that could cause the foreign nurse to feel inadequate and disrespected.

Language differences are also a source of friction between American nurses and foreign nurses. When frictions escalate, foreign nurses may form cliques on a unit. By speaking in their native language and excluding English-speaking nurses, foreign nurses may feel unified, even though they are alienating themselves even further from the rest of the nursing staff (Burner, 1990). English-speaking nurses may believe that they are being talked about by the foreign nurses and thus demand that personnel speak only English on the unit. Foreign nurses, denied the right to speak their own language at work, can feel even more threatened and angry, a feeling that erects further obstacles to transcultural communication.

BRIDGES TO TRANSCULTURAL COMMUNICATION BETWEEN HEALTH CARE PROVIDERS

Although there are many barriers to transcultural communication between health care providers, there are also numerous ways to bridge the gap that separates people from different cultures. This section presents techniques for communicating with team members who have different cultural backgrounds and who may not speak fluent English. We will also explore the important role of the nurse-manager in promoting transcultural communication and averting potential workplace conflicts.

Using Transcultural Communication to Work with Team Members

Nurses have a responsibility to communicate clearly with each other, with physicians, with other health care professionals, and with unlicensed assistive personnel. Murky communications can result in errors that compromise patient care. Thus, nurses must make every effort to communicate clearly.

If you are assigned to work with a nurse or nursing student who is from a different culture and who speaks English as a second language, try these techniques to facilitate communication:

- Recognize that your co-worker probably has an educational background in nursing that is very different from your own.

- Acknowledge that the co-worker's value system and perception of what constitutes "good patient care" may differ from your own.

- Try to assess your co-worker's level of understanding of verbal and written communication. For example, ask a co-worker to explain a physician's order to you in her own words. It also helps to assess a patient with the co-worker and note what terms the person uses to describe the patient's signs and symptoms.

- In communicating with nurses for whom English is a second language, avoid the use of slang terms and regional expressions. For example, Chinese, Japanese, and Filipino nurses may not understand such terms as *piggybacking, doing a double,* or *rigging something to work.*

- Do provide your co-worker with resources such as written procedures and protocols that may help to reinforce your verbal communication.

- Remember to praise your co-worker's competency in technical skills. Inspiring self-confidence in a foreign nurse will make it easier for that person to ask for assistance when needed.

- Appreciate the knowledge that you can gain by working alongside a skilled nurse from another culture. Observe how foreign nurses relate to patients who are from their culture. If you have an open mind, working with foreign co-workers can increase your knowledge of other cultures, enrich your work as a nurse, and foster personal growth (Tilki, Papadopoulos, & Alleyne, 1994).

- When offering constructive criticism, try to use *I statements* instead of *you statements*. For example: "I think that it's very important to address the patient's emotional state when you chart" is better than "You never seem to chart anything about the patient's emotional state."

- If you feel you cannot achieve effective communication with a co-worker, request to work with another person. You do not want to be held accountable for the actions of a nurse with whom you cannot communicate.

- Report to your supervisor if you feel that a nurse or a physician is endangering patients because of language difficulties or different cultural values. Record any problems that occur, and keep a copy of the notes you provide to your supervisor.

Sometimes you may need to work with a foreign physician who is difficult to understand because of language differences or a strong accent. In this case, do not take verbal orders, particularly over the telephone. Even when an order is written, take the time to clarify the order with the physician. Because patients may also find it difficult to understand a foreign physician, you will need to listen carefully and then explain the physician's remarks to the patient.

Another group of health care workers who may have difficulty understanding and speaking English are unlicensed assistive personnel (Walton & Waszkiewiez, 1997). If you are called upon to supervise an unlicensed worker who speaks English as a second language, follow these cautions:

- Delegate appropriate tasks to an unlicensed worker. Match assignments to the worker's level of understanding and skill.

- Do not stop at just delegating an assignment or giving instructions. Instead, make sure that the worker understands your instructions.

- Restate your instructions in clear, concrete terms, and give a demonstration of a procedure if necessary.

- To reduce miscommunication, check for understanding by asking the worker to repeat instructions or do a return demonstration.

- If you are still not satisfied that the communication between the two of you is accurate and effective, repeat your directions and request a repeat demonstration.

- Establish a time frame for the worker to complete assigned tasks. For example, "I want you to feed Mr. Brown before you get Mr. Black out of bed."

- Observe how the worker communicates with patients and performs duties.

- Give workers clear feedback concerning their communication skills and performance of duties. If the worker has performed a procedure incorrectly, offer suggestions for improvement. Demonstrate the procedure as it should be done and ask for a return demonstration.

- If, despite your best efforts, the worker is still unable to perform because of language difficulties, ask your supervisor to work with the person. Again, you do not want to be held responsible for a worker with whom you cannot communicate.

Using Transcultural Communication to Manage a Diverse Staff

To effectively manage a multicultural workforce, a nurse-manager must possess the same high level of cultural sensitivity that is required to successfully care for patients from other cultures. Nurse-managers face many complex issues as they go about their role of supervising nurses and assistive personnel from around the world. The three major issues encountered by nurses in administrative positions are:

1. Clashes in values that arise between foreign nurses and nurses trained in the United States.

2. Language differences that disrupt hospital communications.

3. Tensions and conflicts between staff members that are frequently rooted in racial and cultural differences and that can escalate into lawsuits.

Major tasks of the nurse-manager in a diverse hospital environment include:

1. Helping American nurses acknowledge that nurses from other cultures have values and ideas that are as valuable as their own.

2. Establishing opportunities for improving transcultural communication between staff members.

3. Resolving conflicts between staff members.

4. Resolving tensions between patients and foreign nurses.

5. Helping foreign nurses acclimate to American ways.

Improving Transcultural Communication between Staff Members.
Jamieson and O'Mara (1991) have laid out a broad, six-step program for nurse managers to follow to actively manage a diverse nursing staff:

1. Determine which cultural groups are represented on staff.

2. Understand the organization's values and goals.

3. Decide on what is best for the future of the organization.

4. Analyze present conditions within the organization.

5. Plan ways to reach the desired future state and decide how to manage transitions.

6. Evaluate the results.

More specifically, nurse-managers might consider using the following approaches to diminish tensions between staff members and improve transcultural communication:

- Plan informal meetings for nurses to discuss their cultural values. For example, it may benefit Asian nurses to share with American-born nurses their cultural values concerning respect for authority.

- Provide cultural workshops, and ask knowledgeable individuals to present information about the values, behaviors, and communication patterns of the different cultural groups that are represented on staff.

- Provide classes in English as a second language for foreign nurses who do not speak fluent English or who have difficulty pronouncing words.

- Establish a program for orienting foreign nurses to the hospital or agency (Jein & Harris, 1989). The orientation program should be designed to help newcomers adjust to the new work environment. It is helpful to assign each new nurse to a preceptor who will assist in the orientation process. If possible, the preceptor should be a member of the nurse's cultural group. For maximum benefits, the nurse-manager needs to interview each new nurse every week to find out how that person is adapting to the new hospital culture (Williams & Rodgers, 1993).

- Plan potluck events at which nurses, physicians, and other staff members can socialize and discuss cultural differences informally, in a relaxed environment. For example, each unit in the hospital might plan one potluck event for each shift on a monthly basis. Potluck meals could be planned around a cultural theme: for instance, a traditional Vietnamese dinner one month and a traditional Costa Rican meal the next month (Burner, 1990).

- Confer with specialists in transcultural communication; also hire experts to identify potential areas of conflict and resolve conflicts peacefully before they erupt into legal battles.

Using Transcultural Communication to Resolve Workplace Conflicts. Despite a nurse-manager's best efforts, serious conflicts may still arise between staff members who are from different races and cultures. Conflicts develop in a diverse work environment because people from different cultures are likely to perceive situations differently and thus react to situations in ways that reflect their cultural values. Depending on their culture, people may react to a conflict with anger, denial, silence, distrust, annoyance, or resignation.

Styles of **conflict resolution** are also based in culture. Mainstream American culture emphasizes standing up for your rights, assertiveness, confrontation, and litigation. Traditional Asian cultures and some Native American cultures promote cooperation with others and the avoidance of interpersonal conflicts. Arabs use mediation to settle conflicts and disputes. This method is based on the cultural value of maintaining harmony and balance in life. Mediation helps all parties come to a reasonable compromise while allowing everyone to save face (Jein & Harris, 1989). Because resolutions to conflict differ, nurse-managers must become experts in assessing conflict situations and consciously deciding on the appropriate resolution style (Lowenstein & Glanville, 1995).

In a study of racial and status conflict among nurse administrators, staff nurses, and nursing assistants, the researchers found that employment disputes go through a process before they erupt into a legal dispute (Felstiner, Abel, & Sarat, 1981; Lowenstein & Glanville, 1995). During this process, an **unperceived injurious experience** (unPIE) is transformed into a **perceived injurious experience** (PIE). The steps of this transformation are as follows:

1. *Naming:* At this stage, a person or group recognizes that a particular experience has been injurious. An unPIE is transformed into a PIE.

2. *Blaming:* The PIE is transformed into a grievance, and the injured party blames another person, group, or social entity for the injury.

3. *Claiming:* The injured party now confronts the accused party or social entity and demands remedial action.

4. Once a claim has been made, the claim is either rejected by the institution or resolved, with the two sides coming to an agreement, or it advances into a lawsuit.

Researchers noted that the transformation of unPIEs into PIEs depends on (1) the organizational hierarchy that establishes the norms of expected behavior and also the methods for resolving grievances and (2) the particular characteristics of the individuals who are involved in the legal or labor dispute. Individual characteristics include each person's age, experience, socioeconomic status, personality type, degree of job satisfaction, social position, commitment to cultural values, and perception of prejudice within the organization.

• • • COMMUNICATION CONSIDERATIONS • • •

A knowledgeable nurse-manager can do much to help prevent the transformation of unPIEs into PIEs and the escalation of conflicts into legal disputes. The more nurse-managers understand about the cultures represented in their institution, the better able they will be to resolve conflicts quickly.

Ellis and Hartley (1995) suggest eight steps that a nurse-manager can take to resolve conflicts within a group. The nurse-manager should:

1. Conduct a thorough self-assessment. Managers must ask themselves if they really understand the situation that is at the root of the conflict and if they have any biases or prejudices against the people involved.

2. Analyze the issues or conditions that have created the conflict.

3. Review the analysis, adjust negative attitudes, and try to eliminate any biases that might interfere with solving the problem.

4. Schedule a meeting for all of the people who are involved in the conflict. The manager needs to notify the participants well in advance of the meeting so they start thinking about solutions.

5. Encourage people at the meeting to speak openly about their feelings and viewpoints. Take every suggestion for solving the problem seriously.

6. Summarize all of the solutions that group members have suggested.

7. Help the group narrow the choices for action down to the one or two interventions that appear to be the best.

8. Put together a plan for implementing the choices for action. After the meeting, the manager should send everyone a *written plan of action* and a *time line* that is based on the group's decisions.

Not all conflicts can be resolved in informal group meetings. In a serious legal or labor dispute, the hospital or agency may need to call in experts to negotiate, mediate, or arbitrate a settlement. Negotiation, mediation, and arbitration are *alternative dispute resolution remedies* that organizations use to avoid lengthy, costly, and stressful court hearings (Aiken, 1994; Lowenstein & Glanville, 1995).

- **Negotiation** involves compromising or coming to terms about a specific matter: for example, the terms of a contract. Negotiators help the involved parties solve conflicts by reaching a compromise, in which each party gives in on some points in order to gain certain advantages.

- **Mediation** involves the use of mediators who are neutral third parties. Mediators help the two sides of a conflict identify their needs and come to an agreement.

- **Arbitration** is frequently used to resolve major employer–employee conflicts. The involved parties select a neutral third-party arbitrator who is an expert in the area of contention. The arbitrator hears the case and renders a decision.

Reducing Tensions between Foreign Nurses and Patients. In addition to resolving conflicts between staff members, nurse-managers sometimes need to reduce tensions between patients and foreign nurses. Nurses in administrative positions may face complaints from white patients who are being cared for by nurses who are not native English speakers.

For example, a Filipino nurse whose primary language is Tagalog may place the accent on the second syllable of each word, which is a characteristic speech pattern. The supervisor may need to assure patients that this Filipino nurse is clinically competent, despite her pronunciation of English.

The nurse-manager may also request that nurses speak only English in all public areas of the hospital or agency. The point is that patients may become nervous when they hear nurses speaking a foreign language in their immediate environment. Patients may wonder if their foreign nurses will understand them and provide for their needs (Burner, 1990).

Finally, nurse-managers may want to help some foreign nurses with their nonverbal communication. For example, the nurse-manager could encourage some foreign nurses to increase eye contact with their patients. The manager should explain that such instructions or suggestions are not intended to alter the foreign nurse's culture but rather to improve the nurse's transcultural communication with American patients and health care providers.

REFERENCES

Aiken, T. D., with Catalano, J. T. (1994). *Legal, ethical, and political issues in nursing.* Philadelphia: Davis.

Barbee, E. L. (1993). Racism in U.S. nursing. *Medical Anthropology Quarterly, 7*(4), 346–362.

Brink, P. J. (1990). Cultural diversity in the nursing profession. In J. C. McCluskey & H. K. Grace (Eds.), *Current issues in nursing* (3rd ed.). Boston: Blackwell Scientific.

Burner, O. Y., Cunningham, P., & Hattar, H. S. (1990). Managing a multicultural nurse staff in a multicultural environment. *Journal of Nursing Administration, 20*(6), 30–34.

Ellis, J. R., & Hartley, C. L. (1995). *Managing and coordinating nursing care* (2nd ed.). Philadelphia: Lippincott.

Felstiner, W. L. F., Abel, R. L., & Sarat, A. (1981). The emergence and transformation of disputes: Naming, blaming, claiming. *Law Sociology Review, 15*(34), 631–654.

Giger, J. N., & Davidhizar, R. J. (1996). When the operating room has a multicultural team. *Today's Surgical Nurse, 18*(5), 26–32.

Jamieson, D., & O'Mara, J. (1991). *Managing workforce 2000: Gaining the diversity advantage.* San Francisco: Jossey-Bass.

Jein, R. F., & Harris, B. L. (1989). Cross-cultural conflict: The American nurse manager and a culturally mixed staff. *Journal of the New York State Nurses Association, 20*(2), 16–19.

Lajkowicz, C. (1993). Teaching cultural diversity for the workplace. *Journal of Nursing Education, 32*(5), 235–236.

Lowenstein, A. J., & Glanville, C. (1995). Cultural diversity and conflict in the health care workplace. *Nursing Economics, 13*(4), 203–209.

Spangler, A. (1992). Transcultural care values and practices of Philippine-American nurses. *Journal of Transcultural Nursing, 4*(2), 28–31.

Tilki, M., Papadopoulos, I., & Alleyne, J. (1994). Learning from colleagues of different cultures. *British Journal of Nursing, 3*(21), 1118–1124.

Walton, J. C., & Waszkiewiez, M. (1997). Managing unlicensed assistive personnel: Tips for improving quality outcomes. *Medsurg Nursing, 6*(1), 124–128.

Williams, J., & Rodgers, S. (1993). The multicultural workplace: Preparing preceptors. *Journal of Continuing Education in Nursing, 24*(3), 101–104.

SUGGESTED READINGS

Beamer, L., & Varner, I. (2001). *Intercultural communication in the global workplace.* Boston: McGraw-Hill.

Carr-Rufino, N. (2003). *Managing diversity: People skills for a multicultural workplace.* Needham Heights, MA: Pearson.

Davidhizar, R. E., Dowd, R., Neuman, S., & Giger, J. (1997). Model for cultural diversity in the radiology department. *Radiologic Technology, 68*(3), 233–238.

Gardenswartz, L., & Rowe, A. (1998). *Managing diversity in healthcare.* San Francisco: Jossey-Bass.

Gary, F. A., Sigsby, L. M., & Campbell, D. (1998). Preparing for the 21st century: Diversity in nursing education, research, and practice. *Journal of Professional Nursing, 14*(5), 272–279.

Gropper, R. C. (1996). *Culture and clinical encounter: An intercultural sensitizer for the health professions.* Yarmouth, ME: Intercultural Press.

Harris, L. H., & Tuck, I. (1992). The role of the organization and nurse manager in integrating transcultural concepts into nursing practice. *Holistic Nurse Practitioner, 6*(3), 43–48.

Helman, C. G. (2000). *Culture, health and illness.* Boston: Butterworth Heinemann.

Jandt, F. E. (2003). *An introduction to intercultural communication: Identities in a global community.* Thousand Oaks, CA: Sage.

Jones, M. E., Bond, M. L., & Mancini, M. E. (1998). Developing a culturally competent work force: An opportunity for collaboration. *Journal of Professional Nursing, 15*(5), 180–187.

Judy, R. W., & Amico, C. (1997). *Workforce 2020: Work and workers in the 21st century.* New York: Hudson Institute.

Klopf, D. W. (2001). *Intercultural encounters.* Englewood, CO: Morton Publishers.

Lau, J. (1998). A survey of multicultural awareness among hospital and clinical staff [Letter]. *Journal of Nursing Care Quality, 12*(4), 67–69.

LeBaron, M. (2003). *Bridging cultural conflicts: A new approach for a changing world.* San Francisco: Jossey-Bass.

Leininger, M. (1996). Transcultural nursing administration: An imperative worldwide. *Journal of Transcultural Nursing, 8*(1), 28–33.

Lowenstein, A. J., & Glanville, C. (1991). Transcultural concepts applied to nursing administration. *Journal of Nursing Administration, 21*(3), 13–14.

Rosella, J. D., Regan-Kubinski, M. J., & Albrecht, S. A. (1994). The need for multicultural diversity among health professionals. *Nursing and Health Care, 15*(5), 242–246.

Waxler-Morrison, N., Anderson, J. M., & Richardson, E. (1990). *Cross-cultural caring: A handbook for health professionals.* Vancouver, BC: University of British Columbia Press.

UNIT FIVE
EVALUATION

EVALUATING YOUR TRANSCULTURAL COMMUNICATION SKILLS WITH OTHER HEALTH CARE PROVIDERS

The following exercises will highlight some of the concepts that we discussed in Chapter 15, and they will help you to evaluate the progress that you have made in your interactions with care providers from other cultures.

Exercise One: Evaluating Your Personal Objectives

When you began to study this unit, you were asked to select and write down your personal objectives for learning these new materials. Please review those objectives now.

1. To what extent have you met each objective that you selected from the list of objectives? _____

   _____

   _____

   _____

2. To what extent have you met the personal objectives that you listed?

   _____

   _____

   _____

   _____

3. Have you developed any new objectives since you started this unit?

   _____

   _____

   _____

   _____

Exercise Two: Evaluating Your Personal Responses to Working with Care Providers from Different Cultures

Now that you have studied this unit and you are more aware of your daily interactions with health care providers from other cultures, redo Exercise Two from the self-assessment section of this unit. Select the answer that best describes your point of view *now* that you have completed the unit, and spend some time recording transcultural interactions in your diary.

329

	Agree	Neutral	Disagree
I would rather work with an American nurse than a foreign nurse.	_____	_____	_____
I find it frustrating to work with nurses or physicians who are not proficient in English.	_____	_____	_____
If I thought that a nurse or physician was not fulfilling duties because of cultural or language problems, I would hesitate to report the person for fear that I would be considered prejudiced.	_____	_____	_____
I enjoy working with a skilled foreign nurse. I feel that I can learn a lot from this person.	_____	_____	_____
I like to attend classes and informal meetings where I can learn more about how nurses from other countries are educated.	_____	_____	_____
I do not feel prepared to work with or supervise an unlicensed assistive worker who has some problems with understanding English.	_____	_____	_____

Exercise Three: Reviewing Your *Transcultural Interaction Diary*

1. Have you had any *positive interactions* with health care providers from other cultures? _____

   _____

   What communication skills did you use that helped to make the interaction a positive one? _____

   _____

   Is there anything that you could have done that would have improved your interaction even more? _____

   _____

2. Have you had any *difficult or unsuccessful interactions* with health care providers from other cultures? _____

   What caused the interaction to be difficult or to fail in its intent?

   _____

   What could you have done to prevent the problem?

   _____

Exercise Four: Evaluating Your Readiness for Communicating with Health Care Providers from Other Cultures

Write a brief response to these questions, which are drawn from topics discussed in Chapter 15.

1. List three ways in which language differences can create problems in the workplace.

   a. _____

   b. _____

   c. _____

2. Discuss the attributes of nursing that prevent nurses from openly confronting racism in their profession.

   a. _____

   b. _____

   c. _____

3. When working with a foreign co-worker, what can you do to assess the worker's level of understanding of verbal and written English?

   _____

   _____

   _____

4. Describe at least five techniques that you can use to facilitate communication with a nurse from a foreign country or different culture.

   a. _____

   b. _____

   c. _____

   d. _____

   e. _____

5. What should you do when a foreign physician who is difficult to understand asks you to take a verbal order? _____

   _____

   _____

6. What cautions should you observe when supervising an unlicensed worker who speaks limited English?

   a. _____

   b. _____

   c. _____

   d. _____

   e. _____

   f. _____

7. What are the four stages during which an unperceived injurious experience (unPIE) is transformed into a perceived injurious experience (PIE)?

   a. _____

   b. _____

   c. _____

   d. _____

8. How can conflicts between staff members be resolved without having
   to resort to a lawsuit?

   _____

   _____

   _____

   _____

   _____

   _____

APPENDIX I

Organizations and Agencies

Because this information is of a time-sensitive nature, and URL addresses may change or be deleted, you are encouraged to also conduct your searches by association and/or topic.

PROFESSIONAL ORGANIZATIONS

American Anthropological Association
Society for Linguistic Anthropology (SLA)
Society For Medical Anthropology (SMA)
2200 Wilson Blvd., Suite 600
Arlington, VA 22201
Phone: 703-528-1902
Fax: 703-528-3546
www.aaanet.org/

American Nurses Association
600 Maryland Avenue, SW
Suite 100 West
Washington. DC 20024
Phone: 800-274-4ANA *or*
202-651-7000
Fax: 202-651-7001
www.ana.org

American Psychiatric Nurses Association
1555 Wilson Blvd., Suite 515
Arlington, VA 22209
Phone: 703-243-2443
Fax: 703-243-3390
www.apna.org

Canadian Nurses Association
50 The Driveway
Ottawa, Ontario K2P 1E2
Phone: 800-361-8404 *or*
613-237-2133
Fax: 613-237-3520
www.can-nurses.ca

Council on Nursing and Anthropology
School of Nursing, George Mason University
Fairfax, VA 22030-4444

National Alaska Native American Indian Nurses Association (NANAINA)
3700 Reservoir Road NW
Washington, DC 20057-1107

National Association of Hispanic Nurses
1501 16th Street, NW
Washington, DC 20036
Phone: 202-387-2477
Fax: 202-483-7183
www.thehispanicnurses.org

National Black Nurses Association, Inc.
8630 Fenton Street, Suite 330
Silver Spring, MD 20910
Phone: 301-589-3200
Fax: 301-589-3223
www.nbna.org

National Council for International Health (NCIH)
1701 K Street, NW, Suite 600
Washington, DC 20006
Phone: 202-833-5900
Fax: 202-833-0075
www.ncih.org

Society of Medical Interpreters (SOMI)
c/o Cross-Cultural Health Care Program
Pacific Medical Center
1200 12th Avenue S.
Seattle, WA 98144 *or*
P.O. Box 3304
Seattle, WA 98144
Phone: 206-621-4053
Fax: 206-326-2408
www.sominet.org

Transcultural Nursing Society
36600 Schoolcraft Road
Livonia, MI 48150-1173
Phone: 888-432-5470 *or*
        734-432-5470
Fax: 734-432-5463
www.tcns.org

GOVERNMENT AGENCIES

National Center for Complementary and Alternative Medicine (NCCAM)
NCCAM Clearinghouse
P.O. Box 7923
Gaithersburg, MD 20898
Phone (USA): 888-644-6226
Phone (International): 301-519-3153
TTY (for hearing impaired):
        866-464-3615
Fax: 866-464-3616
info@nccam.nih.gov

Office of Minority Health Resource Center
Office of Minority Health Resource Center
P.O. Box 37337
Washington, DC 20013-7337
Phone: 800-444-6472
Fax: 301-251-2160
www.omhrc.gov

U.S. Department of Commerce, Economics and Statistics Administration
Bureau of the Census
Herbert C. Hoover Building
14th Street and Constitution Avenue NW
Washington, DC 20230
Phone: 202-482-2000
www.census.gov or *www.doc.gov*

U.S. Department of Health and Human Services
U.S. Public Health Service
Indian Health Service, IHS
Parklawn Building
5600 Fishers Lane
Rockville, MD 20857
Phone: 301-443-3593
Fax: 301-443-0507
www.ihs.gov

U.S. Department of Health and Human Services
U.S. Public Health Service
Office of Minority Health, OMH
Rockwall II Building, Suite 1000
5600 Fishers Lane
Rockville, MD 20857
Phone: 800-444-6472 *or*
        301-443-5224
Fax: 301-443-8280
www.hhs.gov

ETHNIC AND MINORITY ORGANIZATIONS AND AGENCIES

American-Arab Antidiscrimination Committee (ADC)
4201 Connecticut Avenue NW
Suite 300
Washington, DC 20008
Phone: 202-244-2990
Fax: 202-244-3196
www.adc.org

American-Arab Relations Committee (AARC)
Box 416
New York, NY 10017
Phone: 516-889-0005

American Civil Liberties Union (ACLU)
125 Broad Street, 18th Floor
New York, NY 10004-2400
www.aclu.org

American Indian Culture Research Center (AICRC)
P.O. Box 98, Blue Cloud Abbey
Marvin, SD 57251-0098
Phone: 605-432-5528
Fax: 605-432-4754
www.bluecloud.org

American Indian Heritage Foundation
6051 Arlington Blvd.
Falls Church, VA 22044
Phone: 202-463-4267
Fax: 703-532-1921
www.indians.org

American Indian Institute
University of Oklahoma
555 Constitution Avenue, Suite 237
Norman, OK 73072-7820
Phone: 405-325-4127
Fax: 405-325-7757

American Jewish Committee
Jacob Blaustein Building
165 E. 56th Street
New York, NY 10022
Phone: 212-751-4000
Fax: 212-838-2120
www.ajc.org

Anti-Defamation League (Seeks to stop defamation of Jewish people)
823 United Nations Plaza
New York, NY 10017
Phone: 212-885-7700
Fax: 212-867-0779
www.adl.org

Asia Society
725 Park Avenue
New York, NY 10021
Phone: 212-288-6400
Fax: 212-517-8315
www.asiasociety.org

Asian and Pacific Islander Partnership for Health
3000 Connecticut Avenue, NW Suite 110
Washington, DC 20008
Phone: 202-986-2393
www.apiph.org

Asian American Legal Defense and Education Fund (AALDEF)
99 Hudson Street, 12th Floor
New York, NY 10013
Phone: 212-966-5932
Fax: 212-966-4303
www.aaldef.org

Cultural Integration Fellowship (CIF)
360 Cumberland Street
San Francisco, CA 94114-2516
Phone: 415-626-2442 *or*
2650 Fulton Street
San Francisco, CA 94118-4063
Phone: 415-386-9590 *or*
415-626-2442
www.culturalintegration.org

Islamic Information Center of America (IICA)
P.O. Box 4052
Des Plaines, IL 60016
Phone: 847-541-8141
Fax: 847-824-8436
www.iica.org

Islamic Information Office
1935 D. Aleo Place
Honolulu, HI 96822
www.iio.org

National Association for the Advancement of Colored People (NAACP)
4805 Mt. Hope Drive
Baltimore, MD 21215
Phone: 410-486-9147 *or*
   877-NAACP-98
Fax: 410-764-7357
NAACP Information Hotline:
   410-521-4939
or
Washington Bureau
1025 Vermont Avenue, NW, Suite 1120
Washington, DC 20005
Phone: 202-638-2269
www.naacp.org

National Latina Health Network (NLHN)
P.O. Box 7567
Oakland, CA 94601
Phone: 510-534-1362
Fax: 510-534-1364
www.nationallatinahealthnetwork.com

National Urban League (NUL)
120 Wall Street
New York, NY 10005
Phone: 212-558-5300
Fax: 212-558-5332
www.nul.org

INTERNATIONAL AGENCIES

Global Health Council
1701 K Street, NW, Suite 600
Washington, DC 20006-1503
Phone: 202-833-5900
Fax: 202-833-0075
E-mail: *ghc@globalhealth.org* or
www.globalhealth.org

International Council of Nurses (ICN)
3, place Jean Marteau
1201 Geneva, Switzerland
Fax: 41-22-9080101
Phone: 41-22-9080100
www.icn@icn.ch

National Council for International Health (NCIH)
1701 K Street, NW, Suite 600
Washington, DC 20006
Phone: 202-833-5900
Fax: 202-833-0075
www.ncih.org

Pan American Health Organization
Nursing Section, Health Services Division
525 23rd Street, NW
Washington, DC 20037
Phone: 202-974-3000
Fax: 202-338-3663
www.paho.org

Project HOPE
The People to People Health Foundation, Inc.
Health Sciences Education Center, Carter Hall
Milkwood, VA 22646
Phone: 800-544-4673 *or*
   540-837-2100
Fax: 540-837-1813
www.projhope.org

World Health Organization (WHO)
Headquarters:
Avenue Appia 20
1211 Geneva 27
Switzerland
Phone: 41-22-791-21-11
Regional Office:
525 23rd Street NW
Washington, DC 20037-2832
Phone: 202-974-3000
Fax: 202-974-3663
www.who.org

REFUGEE CENTERS AND PROGRAMS

Central American Refugee Center (CARECEN)
3112 Mount Pleasant Street NW
Washington, DC 20010
Phone: 202-328-9799
Fax: 202-328-2300 *or*
91 N. Franklin Street
Hempstead, NY 11550
Phone: 516-489-8330

Haitian Refugee Center (HRC)
119 NE 54th Street
Miami, FL 33137
Phone: 305-757-8538
Fax: 305-758-2444

Refugee Policy Group (RPG)
1424 16th Street NW, Suite 401
Washington, DC 20036-2211
Phone: 202-387-3015
Fax: 202-667-5034

United States Committee for Refugees (USCR)
1717 Massachusetts Avenue NW, Suite 701
Washington, DC 20036
Phone: 202-347-3507
Fax: 202-347-3418
www.irsa-uscr.org

TELEPHONE INFORMATION LINES

Centers for Disease Control and Prevention
Immunizations and Vaccinations Information Hotline
800-232-2522
www.cdc.gov

Immigration and Naturalization Service (INS)
Toll-free request phone number for INS forms: 800-870-FORM (3676)
www.ins.usdoj.gov

APPENDIX II

Annotated List of Suggested Books and Films with a Transcultural Theme

FICTION

Blu's Hanging by Ann Yamanaka (1997), a drama set in the author's native Hawaii, depicts the harrowing lives of three destitute children who are left to survive on the Island of Molokai after their mother's death. Yamanaka, a Japanese American writer, has won awards for her lyrical poems and realistic novels about Hawaiian life.

Breath, Eyes, Memory by Edwidge Danticat (1994) is the story of Sophie, a young girl who grows up in Haiti, spends a rebellious adolescence in New York City, and then returns to Haiti to reconcile with her mother. This powerful debut novel by Haitian author Danticat has been compared with the early novels of black Nobel Laureate Toni Morrison.

In Broken WigWag by Suchi Asano (1997) tells the story of Satomi, a Japanese expatriate who has been living for eight years in a cramped apartment in lower Manhattan. Satomi longs for a more fulfilling life but does not know where to find it. This novel provides an interesting look into the American Japanese community and the everyday lives of young Japanese women.

Dark Blue Suit and Other Stories by Peter Bacho (1997) contains a dozen semi-autobiographical stories that take place in the Filipino community of Seattle, Washington. Several of the stories describe Bacho's pursuit of the art of boxing at the "Bruce Lee school" as a way for him to gain respect—"the most precious currency of the poor and colored."

Eating Chinese Food Naked by Mei Ng (1998) is a coming-of-age story about Ruby Lee, a Chinese, Columbia University graduate who returns home to her parents, who work and live in a laundry in Queens, New York. The novel explores the problems that Ruby experiences as she tries to reconcile contemporary American ways with the traditional cultural values of her parents.

Fragile Night by Stella Pope Duarte (1997) is a collection of fifteen short slice-of-life stories about life in the barrio. Her stories describe the lives of long-suffering Latina women, who in the Latino cultural tradition, feel that they must put up with their husbands' infidelities and abuse.

Go Tell It on the Mountain by James Baldwin (1953), a first novel, was the largely autobiographical work that established Baldwin as a writer. In addition to his essays, Baldwin wrote other influential novels including *Giovanni's Room, Another*

Country, and *Tell Me How Long the Train's Been Gone*. Baldwin was deeply involved in the civil rights movement, and his writings focused on the racism that blacks face in America.

Honey, Hush!: An Anthology of African American Women's Humor edited by Daryl Cumber Dance (1997), covers 200 years of black women's biting humor and satire that ranges from slave narratives to contemporary fiction by Terry McMillan, author of *Waiting to Exhale* and *How Stella Got Her Groove Back*.

The Joy Luck Club by Amy Tan (1989) is a collection of sixteen interconnected stories that explore the complex transcultural relationships between four mothers who are Chinese immigrants born before World War II and their four American-born daughters, who are first-generation Californians. *The Joy Luck Club* was released as a motion picture in 1993.

Krik? Krak! by Edwidge Danticat (1996) is a collection of short fiction that depicts the difficulties and tragedies that are a part of everyday life in the author's war-torn homeland of Haiti. These stories also give the reader insight into the myths and folklore that have evolved through generations of Haitians.

A Lesson before Dying by Ernest Gaines (1993) is set in rural Louisiana in 1948. This is the story of a young black man who is falsely accused by the white community and who finds dignity as he faces the electric chair for a robbery and murder that he did not commit. In this and other novels, Gaines stresses the need for black men to "stand tall" and face injustice and adversity with courage.

The Lone Ranger and Tonto Fist Fight in Heaven by Sherman Alexie (1995) is a collection of short stories about Native Americans that was used as the basis for the film *Smoke Signals*. This film, by and about young Native Americans, describes the journey of two young men from the reservation to Phoenix, Arizona, to claim one of the father's ashes.

Medicine of the Cherokee by J. T. Garrett and Michael Garrett (1996), both teachers of Indian medicine, describes the holistic medicine of the Cherokee Nation.

Midnight Sandwiches and the Mariposa Express by Beatriz Rivera (1997) is a witty first novel that tells the story of Cuban immigrant Trish Izquierdo, who is a town councilwoman in a fictitious New Jersey town. The Mariposa Express is the town's popular cafeteria, where Trish meets with other primarily Hispanic characters to discuss the latest town gossip and political scandals.

Night Talk by Elizabeth Cox (1997) opens during the racially turbulent 1950s and depicts the growing friendship between two adolescent girls—one the daughter of a white research biologist and the other the daughter of a black domestic who works for the white family. The "night talks" between the girls, who share a bedroom, and later their letters to each other, form a deeply personal basis for describing the drama of the civil rights movement.

Ourselves among Others: Cross-Cultural Readings for Writers (3rd edition) by Carol J. Verburg (1994) is an anthology of cross-cultural short stories, memoirs, and essays by authors from all over the world. Among the authors are such highly regarded writers as Octavio Paz, Margaret Atwood, Günter Grass, Carlos Fuentes, and Simone de Beauvoir.

Paradise by Toni Morrison (1998), the author's seventh novel, takes place between the 1970s and late 1980s and is set outside of the all-black town of Ruby, Oklahoma. The book describes the lives of a group of women who live in an old house called The Convent. It also focuses on generational conflicts, racial conflicts, and the elusive meaning of paradise. The Nobel Prize–winning author has also written *The Bluest Eye, Son of Solomon*, and *Beloved* among other novels.

Short Fiction by Hispanic Writers of the United States edited by Nicolas Kanellos (1993) contains Puerto Rican, Cuban American, and Mexican American short fiction in which authors tell stories about Hispanic life in the United States.

Snow Falling on Cedars by David Guterson (1995) is a complex transcultural drama that on one level recounts the trial of Kubuo Miyamoto, a Japanese American who is accused of murdering a local fisherman on San Piedro Island in Washington State. On a deeper level, the novel addresses the tragic fate of the Japanese residents of San Piedro Island who were sent into exile during World War II.

Sweetbitter: A Novel by Reginald Gibbons (1994) is a turn-of-the-century tale set in East Texas. Gibbons tells the story of Reuben S. Sweetbitter, a young half-Choctaw, half-white man who has lost contact with his Choctaw roots. The novel describes Sweetbitter's attempts to find his place in the world, his forbidden love relationship with a young white woman, and his flight with her to a place where they hope to find peace and acceptance.

A ***Treasury of African-American Christmas Stories*** compiled and edited by Bettye Collier-Thomas (1997), studies black culture at the beginning of the twentieth century through short stories, poetry, and newspaper and magazine stories. This anthology also provides short biographies of the authors, describing each author's contribution to black literature, black culture, and American society.

NONFICTION

Angela's Ashes by Frank McCourt (1996) is the gritty childhood memoir of the author's Irish childhood. McCourt describes how he grew up poor and miserable in the slums of Limerick, with a drunken father and a mother named Angela, who desperately tried to hold her starving family together.

James Baldwin: Collected Essays edited by Toni Morrison (1998) compiles Baldwin's influential essays that helped to expose the polarization of blacks and whites in America. This massive anthology contains several essay collections including *Notes of a Native Son* (1955), *Nobody Knows My Name* (1961), *The Fire Next Time* (1963), *No Name in the Street* (1972), *The Devil Finds Work* (1976), and a group of articles and interviews called *The Price of the Ticket* (1985), which was published two years before Baldwin's death from cancer.

Beyond the Godfather: Italian American Writers on the Real Italian American Experience edited by A. Kenneth Ciongoli and Jay Parini (1997) is a collection of twenty-three essays on Italian American culture. The essays are divided into personal reflections on life as an Italian American, the Italian American literary tradition, and the Italian American heritage.

Bloodlines: Odyssey of a Native Daughter by Janet Campbell (1998) contains the author's family history in seven autobiographical essays. Campbell is a member of the Coeur d'Alene tribe of northern Idaho.

The Children by David Halberstam (1998) chronicles the lives of eight idealistic young black college students who evolved into leaders of the civil rights movement. The story covers five years, beginning with sit-ins in 1960 and ending with the passage of the Voting Rights Act of 1965.

A Country of Strangers: Blacks and Whites in America by David K. Shipler (1997) is a record of the in-depth interviews of this former *New York Times* correspondent with hundreds of people across the United States. From his interviews, Shipler concluded that black Americans and white Americans have little knowledge or understanding of each other's lives.

A Culture of Emotions: A Cultural Competence and Diversity Training Program produced by Harriet Koskoff (2002) is a sixty-minute video that is an excellent introduction for professionals wishing to learn cultural competence and diversity skills in academic, medical, and psychiatric settings. Although the tape is well grounded by establishing a strong theoretical foundation in each of its sections, it is clinically very practical for professionals working with a broad spectrum of patients in culturally diverse settings. This tape features didactic interviews and skill-building exercises with distinguished researchers and clinicians who are experienced in both theoretical and practical areas of cultural psychiatry. The focus of the tape is on building the skills necessary to use DSM IV in a culturally competent way in evaluation and treatment. The tape provides a conceptual bridge between Euro-Western diagnostic concepts, categories, and etiological explanations of illness and traditional views of health, disease, and pathology in diverse cultural groups from around the world.

Daughters of Kings: Growing Up as a Jewish Woman in America edited by Leslie Brody (1997) is a collection of academic essays written by thirteen fellows of the Bunting Institute at Radcliffe College, which explores the topics of Jewish heritage and Jewish identity. Authors from many ethnic backgrounds describe their experiences either as Jewish women or as non-Jewish women who are living and working in a Jewish community.

Death and Dying in Central Appalachia: Changing Attitudes and Practices by James K. Crissman (1994) uses photographs, archival sources, and interviews with over 400 mountain dwellers to explore the rituals associated with death, dying, and funeral customs in the Appalachian sections of Tennessee, Virginia, Kentucky, North Carolina, and West Virginia.

Double Burden: Black Women and Everyday Racism by Yanick St. Jean and Joe R. Feagin (1998) presents a study based on interviews and focus groups with 200 black women. In the book, the black women respondents describe their feelings of being "physically, morally, and spiritually stigmatized by a dominant culture."

The Famine Ships: The Irish Exodus to America by Edward Laxton (1998) is an illustrated chronicle of the experiences of the 1 million Irish immigrants who fled from their miserable lives in Ireland in the hope of finding peace and prosperity in America.

Growing Up Chicana/o: An Anthology edited by Tiffany Ana Lopez (1993) contains the writings of twenty authors. Each author describes the experience of being a child who grows up caught between rich Hispanic traditions and the need to assimilate into mainstream American culture.

Growing Up Native American: An Anthology edited by Patricia Riley (1993) contains the essays and short stories of twenty-two authors whose writings span the years from the nineteenth century to the 1990s. Each of these authors explore the many challenges that are faced by Native American youths who are coming of age in the United States and Canada.

Heart of a Woman by Maya Angelou (1981) is the fourth volume of the acclaimed author's autobiography. In this book, Angelou looks back on her life as a black woman in America, her civil rights work with Martin Luther King Jr., and her fascinating encounters with such famous blacks as Billie Holiday and Malcolm X.

Lay My Burden Down by Alvin Pouissant and Amy Alexander (2000) describes the issue of mental health problems and suicide among African Americans. Theories are presented as well as case studies for which solutions are proposed.

Leaving Deep Water: The Lives of Asian American Women at the Crossroads of Two Cultures by Claire S. Chow (1998) presents Chow's study of racial identity; her interviews with 120 primarily middle-class, Asian American women; and personal narrative. A psychotherapist, Chow learned that, like herself, some of the women felt confused about their racial identity, while others were proud of their Asian heritage. Respondents who had grown up in racially integrated Hawaii had the fewest identity problems.

Makes Me Wanna Holler: A Young Black Man in America by Nathan McCall (1994) is a first-person account of a young black man who is from a decent family but who is nevertheless lured into a life of crime and violence. At nineteen, McCall is sentenced to twelve years in prison for robbing a fast-food joint. In prison, McCall is exposed to books, then completes college while on parole, and then finally becomes a successful newspaper man on the *Washington Post*.

The Maria Paradox: How Latinas Can Merge Old World Traditions with New World Self-Esteem by Rosa Maria Gil and Carmen Inoa Vazquez (1996) asks this question: How can a Hispanic woman empower herself with North American ways without giving up the valued Latin tradition that the female role is one of submission to male authority? To answer this question, the authors (both Latina psychotherapists) present Hispanic women with methods for balancing family and career demands, creating a sense of partnership within a traditional marriage, and standing up for their own feelings and rights.

Miners and Medicine: West Virginia Memories by Claude A. Frazier, MD (1992) recalls Dr. Frazier's memories of the coal camps of Appalachia where his father was a camp doctor. The book describes the horrific health problems and hazardous, diseased working environment faced by the coal miners before the United Mine Workers of America promoted better working conditions and medical care.

The Nawal El Saadawi Reader: Selected Essays, 1970–1996 by Nawal el Saadawi (1997) is a collection of twenty-three essays written by a woman who is considered by some to be the leading authority on the status of women in the Arab world. Her essays cover a variety of topics ranging from women's health to the impact of Islamic fundamentalism on Arab women's movement toward political change.

Ono Ono Girl's Hula by Carolyn Lei-lanilau (1997) is a collection of humorous but angry short essays that address the problems inherent in being a person of mixed race in America. Lei-lanilau, a winner of the American Book Award for poetry, was raised in Hawaii by her Chinese mother and Hawaiian Turkish father before coming to the mainland United States.

The Rez Road Follies: Canoes, Casinos, Computers, and Birch Baskets by Jim Northrup (1997) humorously describes life on an Indian reservation and in a federal boarding school for young Native Americans, as experienced by Northrup—a member of the Anishinaabe tribe, a newspaper columnist, and the author of *Walking the Rez Road*. With sadness and humor, Northrop recalls his days at the federal school, where he was taught about the ways of white society or, in his words, the "immigrant community."

In Search of the Racial Frontier: African Americans in the American West by Quintard Taylor (1998) covers the era from the early sixteenth century to the present. The book documents how black Westerners struggled to integrate themselves into the larger society while working as doctors, lawyers, schoolteachers, newspaper editors, restaurant owners, barbershop owners, newspaper editors, waiters, and cooks.

Why Are All the Black Kids Sitting Together in the Cafeteria? by Beverly Daniel Tatum (2003) is a book that explains the intricacy and development of cultural value systems for racial groups and racial identity. Racial interactions and barriers are also discussed.

Wisdom's Daughters: Conversations with Women Elders of Native America written and photographed by Steve Wall (1994) combines more than 100 photographs with the words of Native American women elders to paint a vivid portrait of a unified, harmonious philosophy of life.

With a Whoop and a Holler: A Bushel of Lore from Way Down South by Nancy Van Laan (1998) is a collection of fresh and funny Southern folklore, homespun tales, outlandish rhythms and riddles, old-time superstitions, and ribald colloquialisms drawn from the bayous of Alabama, the mountains of Appalachia, and the intriguing culture of the deep South.

FILMS

Alamo Bay (1985) is a story that takes place in the late 1970s. Vietnamese refugees come to the Gulf Coast of Texas in hopes of building a new life in America. Instead, to their horror, the refugees come face to face with racist American fishermen and Ku Klux Klan members.

The Defiant Ones (1958) This Academy Award–winning film tells the story of two convicts—one black and one white—who escape from a Southern prison. Shackled together, the convicts initially hate and distrust each other but must learn to work together in order to survive. As the two men deal with escalating difficulties, they develop a respect for each other.

Driving Miss Daisy (1990) is based on a Pulitzer Prize–winning play by Alfred Uhry. This film explores the unconventional, twenty-five-year relationship between Miss Daisy—a strong-willed, Southern, Jewish widow—and her chauffeur, Hoke

Colburn—an illiterate, dignified, black widower. The film winds its way through many small adventures, little arguments, and reconciliations. In the end, when Miss Daisy is visited by Hoke in the nursing home, she finally realizes that despite their differences, her chauffeur is truly her best friend.

Falling Down (1993) is a film in which a divorced white man who has lost his job as a defense worker, as well as the right to see his little daughter on her birthday, "cracks up" under the strain. Going on a rampage in East Los Angeles, this disenfranchised white male who feels violated and enraged, violently confronts a Korean grocery store owner, Mexican gang members, and a Neo-Nazi. Finally, he brings about his own death during a shoot-out with a police detective.

Grand Avenue (Made for Cable, 1996) This slice-of-life made-for-television movie dramatizes the traumatic changes faced by a Native American mother and her children, who leave the reservation for a new life in an urban neighborhood. The family tries to start life over in a California town, only to be threatened by gangs and almost destroyed by neighborhood violence.

Heaven and Earth (1993) Preceded by *Platoon* (1986) and *Born on the Fourth of July* (1989), this is the third film in a trilogy about Vietnam by director Oliver Stone. The story follows the unhappy life of Le Ly, a young Vietnamese woman who marries an American Marine sergeant and returns home with him to California. She is unable to cope with her emotionally disturbed husband, and Le Ly's life and marriage fall apart because of cultural clashes and postwar stress.

The Joy Luck Club (1993) Based on the successful 1989 novel by Amy Tan, this film blends eight stories and numerous flashbacks to portray the turbulent lives of four brave Chinese women who survived China's pre-World War II, male-dominated culture. The film depicts the women's emigration to the United States, and it explores their complex relationships with their four American-born daughters.

Lone Star (1996) Hispanics, blacks, and Anglos attempt to live together in a Texas border town that was once dominated by a cruel, racist, and murderous white sheriff. This film dramatizes both the investigation of a forty-year-old murder mystery and the love between the sheriff's son and the Mexican woman with whom he grew up.

Mi Familia (*My Family*, 1995) With a time frame that stretches from the 1920s to the present, *Mi Familia* traces the struggles of a Mexican American family who call East Los Angeles home. A strong religious faith and a deep sense of togetherness help family members survive discrimination, racism, deportation, imprisonment, and the tragic death of a son.

Mississippi Masala (1992) This romantic comedy draws its title from its location (a small town in Mississippi) and masala, which is a blending of hot, multicolored, Indian spices. The story is about the transcultural love affair between Demetrius, a young black Mississippian, and Mina, a young woman from Uganda, and the heat that their relationship generates in this traditional Southern community.

Mi Vita Loca (*My Crazy Life*, 1994) This offbeat, independent film explores life among the Latina girl gangs in Echo Park, a potentially violent ethnic area of Los Angeles. The writer-director, Allison Anders, lived in this troubled neighborhood for several years and spent time with the "homegirls" and their male friends. Her movie about Sad Girl and Mousie and the love they jealously share with a neighborhood drug dealer gives the viewer a glimpse into the hopelessness of inner-city life.

Mr. and Mrs. Loving (1996) This is the true story of a working-class Southern couple, Mr. and Mrs. Loving, who are driven out of their native state of Virginia because their mixed marriage violates antimiscegenation laws. The Lovings took their case to the U.S. Supreme Court, which abolished antimiscegenation laws in the early 1960s.

El Norte (1983) A Guatemalan brother and sister make a long and dangerous journey from their violence-torn homeland to the United States, which they call *El Norte*. Once in Los Angeles, the young people, filled with hope, attempt to start new lives only to discover fresh obstacles and prejudices. One of the most unforgettable scenes in the film is when the sister is attacked and bitten by rats, as she and her brother fight their way across the border through subterranean tunnels.

Not in This Town (1997) This is the true-life story of a Jewish family who stands up to a vicious Neo-Nazi clan in Billings, Montana. The resulting conflict from this ethnic confrontation creates an upheaval that affects the entire community.

A Price above Rubies (1998) An ultra-Orthodox Jewish (Hasidic) wife who lives in New York City discovers that she can no longer play the traditional and sexually suppressed role expected of women in a patriarchal society. At first, the unhappy wife looks for love with her brother-in-law, who is a jeweler, but then finds sexual fulfillment with a Puerto Rican artist. The title, *A Price above Rubies*, is drawn from a biblical parable.

Selena (1997) A biographical drama, this film presents the short life of Selena Quintanilla Perez, a charismatic Mexican American Tejano singer. Selena was murdered in 1995 at the age of 23 by an ex-fan-club president. The movie contains many memorable scenes that portray life within Selena's loving, close-knit, and supportive Mexican American family. The film also depicts the prejudice and condescending attitudes that confront Mexican Americans. For example, when Selena enters a stylish dress shop and begins to try on clothes, the salesperson automatically assumes that Selena (who is by now very wealthy) cannot afford to buy clothes in her shop because she is Mexican American.

Smoke Signals (1998) Based on *The Lone Ranger and Tonto Fist Fight in Heaven*, a 1995 collection of short stories by Sherman Alexie, *Smoke Signals* was written, directed, and produced by Native Americans. It tells about the journey of two young Native American men from the reservation to Phoenix, Arizona, to claim one of the father's ashes. *Smoke Signals* won a major prize at the prestigious Sundance Film Festival.

A Stranger among Us (1992) is a transcultural police drama placed in Brooklyn. A policewoman goes to live in a close-knit Hasidic Jewish community, where she searches for the "insider" who has murdered a community member. In the course of infiltrating this community, the brash, tough policewoman dons modest Hasidic female clothing, observes traditional dietary and religious customs, and even falls in love with a devout Hasidic scholar.

Sunchaser (1996) A cultural clash arises when a privileged white male oncologist is forced to treat a dying half-Navajo called Blue, who is a convicted murderer. Blue forces the doctor to drive him to a mountaintop in Arizona where he can seek the help of a medicine man and cure his cancer by swimming in a magical, healing lake. As the physician and the young Navajo cross the desert together in search of spiritual healing, they eventually bond and come to see each other in a new light.

Witness (1985) A complex film with many layers, *Witness* is a detective story, a love story, and a transcultural portrait of the dramatic differences between Amish and mainstream American values. A young Amish boy on a journey with his mother witnesses a murder. Through a series of misadventures, the police detective assigned to the case is wounded, and the Amish community takes him in and hides him from the gunman. The young mother nurses the detective back to health, and, during this process, the two fall in love. The young woman is warned by her alarmed father that she risks being shunned by the community if she continues her involvement with the detective. By the end of the film, the detective has solved the murder mystery, and he sadly leaves the Amish woman he loves, and the unyielding traditions of the Amish community, behind him.

INDEX

role of, 314–316
three types of racism, 313
workforce conditions, 310
Nursing
as a culture, 100
and cultural competence, 46
educational differences, 316–317
obligation to care, 315
and racism, 81–82, 313
ritual behavior, 85, 86
staff responsibilities, 314
as subculture, 23, 98–100
Nursing diagnoses
cultural bias, 229–230
culturally appropriate, 235–237
development, 223–225
NANDA sample, 226–228
promoting culturally appropriate, 237–238
taxonomy development, 224
Nutrition, cultural assessment, 207

O
Observer as participant, 125, 130–135
Obstacles, care plan, 259–260
Occupation, cultural assessment, 209
Office for Civil Rights (OCR), medical interpreter services, 181
Old Order Amish, cultural values, 34–35
Oral language, communication, 14
Organizational supports, CLAS theme, 51, 52–53
Orientation, cultural assessment, 207
Orientation phase, described, 143, 145
Orthodox Jews, 40

P
Pain
chemical control theory, 284
defined, 279
diary, 250
Filipino values, 37
gate control theory, 283
management of, 283
responses to, 279–282
universality of, 279
Pain threshold, defined, 279

Pain tolerance, defined, 279
Paraphrasing, techniques, 155
Participant as observer, 125–126, 135–136
Participant observation (PO)
cultural understanding, 162–163
described 122–125
four phases of, 125–126
interviewing, described 137–138
Patient
care plan preferences, 258
and foreign nurses, 325
as lay culture, 169
learning style, 265
multiple realities, 163
readiness to learn, 263–264
as subculture, 100–101
Patient Self-Determination Act (PSDA), requirements, 257
Perceived injurious experience, 323
Perception
as barrier, 78, 88–89, 162, 169–171
pain response, 279
Personal care, 209
Personal space
patient communication, 157
Western culture, 72
Perspective, as barrier, 169
Pharmacologic therapy
alternative system, 65
pain management, 283
Physical therapy, pain management, 283
Pilipino, Filipino languages, 36
Pogrom (anti-Jewish riot), 40
Policy makers, CLAS standards, 51
Popular health care system, 63, 64–65
Population categories
census figures, 16
diversity within, 18
Posture, nonverbal standards, 73
Poverty, population distribution, 32–33
Powerlessness, diagnosis, 230, 233
Preinteraction phase, described, 143–144
Preoccupation, grief, 290
Process recording, defined, 116